T0035691

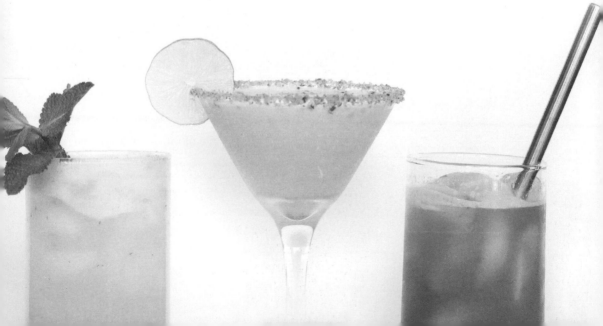

DRINKING
FOR TWO

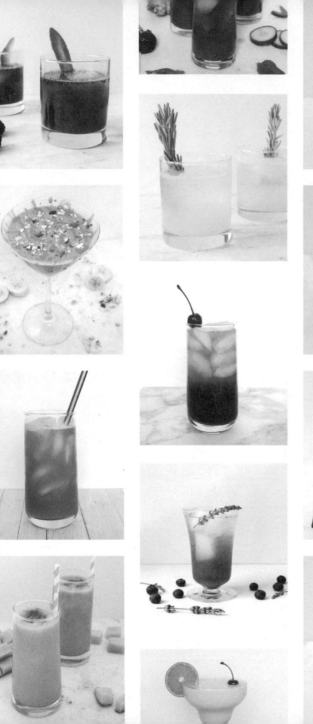
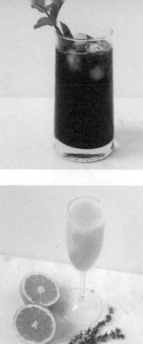
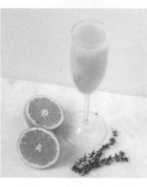
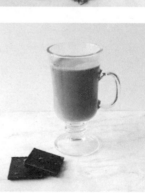
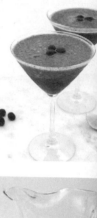
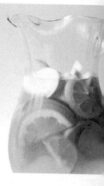
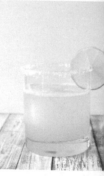

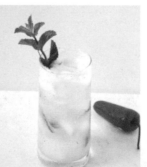

DRINKING FOR TWO

NUTRITIOUS MOCKTAILS
FOR THE MOM-TO-BE

WRITTEN BY

DIANA LICALZI MALDONADO, MS, RDN

KERRY BENSON, MS, RDN

Photography by Kerry Benson & Diana Licalzi Maldonado

Illustrations & Cover Design by Amanda Hudson

Design by Amy Sly

ISBN 978-1944515829

Printed in Colombia

15 14 13 12 11 10 9 8 7

DISCLAIMER:
This book is for informational and educational purposes. This book is not intended to be a substitute for the medical advice of a licensed physician. The reader should consult with his or her doctor in any matters relating to her/his health.

The information in this book is not intended to treat, diagnose, cure, or prevent disease. This book is not sponsored or endorsed by any organization or company. The information included in this book is based on experience and research done by the authors. Neither the publisher nor the authors accept any liability of any kind for any damages caused, directly or indirectly, from the use of the information in this book.

Copyright © Kerry Benson & Diana Licalzi Maldonado

Published by Blue Star Press
PO Box 8835, Bend, OR 97708
contact@bluestarpress.com
www.bluestarpress.com

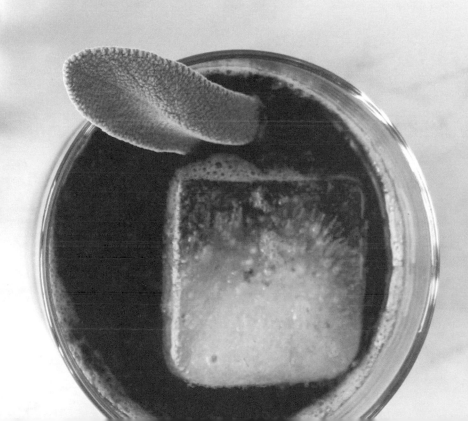

✦

WE ARE IMMENSELY GRATEFUL TO OUR FRIENDS AND FAMILY
FOR THEIR INPUT AND ENCOURAGEMENT THROUGHOUT THE
DEVELOPMENT OF THIS BOOK. THIS WOULD NOT HAVE BEEN
POSSIBLE WITHOUT YOUR SUPPORT AND TASTE BUDS, AND
WE DEDICATE THIS BOOK TO YOU.

Kerry & Diana

✦

DRINKING FOR TWO
CONTENTS

PREFACE

———————————————————————◆———————————————————————

Diana and Kerry met serendipitously while volunteering for an after-school program that teaches cooking classes at a local elementary school in Boston. They were fast friends: they studied together, worked out together, and even played matchmaker for each other. Now, they've written a book together!

When they met in 2015, they had just started their first semester at the Tufts University Friedman School of Nutrition Science & Policy, the first nutrition graduate school in North America and one of the most respected nutrition institutions in the world. Here's a little background on their unique and formative experiences with nutrition and their journeys to pursuing their dream job as registered dietitians:

With a Puerto Rican mother and an Italian father, Diana was raised and immersed in two deeply rooted cultures that hold food central in their traditions. Diana grew up in Puerto Rico, where she noted the poor eating habits on the island and recognized that culture, barriers to education, and a relatively weak economy conspired against proper nutrition. As a registered dietitian with a familiarity of Latin culture, Diana knew she could make a meaningful difference in the lives and health of Hispanics. Diana earned a Master's in Nutrition Science and Policy at Tufts, and entered the Dietetic Internship at UC San Diego Health, where she completed her clinically-focused supervised practice in several different fields within nutrition including diabetes, cardiology, oncology, and weight management. After successfully passing the Registered Dietitian Examination in 2018, Diana launched a private practice offering nutrition consultations to individuals in both English and Spanish focusing primarily on diabetes and weight management.

Kerry worked in an alcohol research lab at the University of Delaware for more than six years while earning Bachelor's and Master's in Neuroscience degrees. Kerry was a competitive figure skater growing up. Though proper nutrition was essential to her training, she struggled with disordered eating and body image for many years. Despite the omnipresence of nutrition in her life, Kerry did not appreciate its influence or importance to health until after she stopped skating. Her desire to become a registered dietitian stems from her personal journey

———————————————————————◆———————————————————————

A registered dietitian nutritionist (RD or RDN) is a nutrition expert who is credentialed by the Commission on Dietetic Registration, a body of the Academy of Nutrition and Dietetics (AND). To become an RDN, one must complete rigorous coursework at an accredited institution and more than 1200 hours of supervised practice, in addition to passing a national exam. The education is comprehensive, covering food science to nutrient metabolism to epidemiology and statistics. RDNs must complete continuing education to maintain their credentials and to keep up with current research. Note that not all "nutritionists" are RDNs.

with nutrition, which gives her an appreciation of the power of food to harm and to heal. Kerry always hoped to pursue a career that would allow her to directly impact people's lives, and dietetics represents the perfect blend of science, people, and food. Her experiences in the neuroscience lab sparked her interest in early life experiences and pregnancy and fueled her desire to work in maternal-infant nutrition as a future dietitian.

Though they were pursuing different degrees at Tufts (Diana earned a Master's in Nutrition Science and Policy, and Kerry received her Master's in Nutritional Epidemiology), they shared the same end goal: to become a registered dietitian. Now both Kerry and Diana are practicing RDNs, having completed their dietetic internships and passed the national exam. It was important for them to pursue this credential so that they can practice as trained and respected healthcare professionals. They were fortunate enough to have had the opportunity to simultaneously complete the coursework necessary to become a dietitian while attaining graduate-level degrees. This gave them additional experience and education that will support their career goals and will also allow them to stay competitive: all rising dietitians will be required to get a master's degree starting in 2024.

This book truly represents the fruits of their personal friendship and fusion of their professional strengths, combining Diana's knack for recipe development, Kerry's interest in nutrition during pregnancy, and their shared love of food, nutrition education, and a whole food, plant-based approach to eating. They were struck by the fact that very few books on nutrition in pregnancy, including cookbooks, provide alternatives to alcoholic beverages or drink recipes beyond smoothies—even though they all say that alcohol should be avoided! What's more, mocktails and their alcoholic counterparts are often loaded with sugar, syrup, and other undesirable ingredients. Seltzer water is great, especially with all of the fun flavors out there, but will that quench your thirst for a margarita on Taco Tuesday? With all of this in mind, Diana and Kerry set out to fill the gap and develop recipes that are not only free of alcohol but nutritious and flavorful.

This book opens with a pregnancy-focused nutrition primer but also includes information relevant to women who are hoping to conceive, women who are postpartum, and even men. In Chapter 2, Kerry and Diana describe the tools and tricks of the "mocktail" trade. They are not expert mixologists, and they do not expect you to be either! With this in mind, they have kept the ingredients and methods as simple as possible.

Then they share extensively tested beverage recipes. While all of the recipes are plant-based, they can easily be adapted to accommodate any dietary preferences or restrictions. They recommend only ingredients that are safe for you and your baby. These drinks are made with everyday items that you can find at your local food store, and on the recipe pages you will see suggestions for using leftover ingredients to keep food waste to a minimum. Throughout the book, recipes highlight benefits of various ingredients, particularly those that help manage common pregnancy symptoms like nausea and swelling. These recipes are suitable for anyone looking to eliminate alcohol without feeling left out at parties and events—in fact, if you start serving these drinks, people will be coming to YOU for drink-spiration. This book is truly a labor of love, and Kerry and Diana hope you enjoy the mocktails as much as they do. Cheers!

1

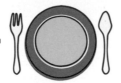

NUTRITION
PRIMER

M ost of us know that how we eat affects our health but having a baby on board or thinking about trying to get pregnant can motivate us to be more proactive about taking care of ourselves and nourishing our bodies. It is never too early—or too late—to start making positive changes to improve your health and do right by yourself and your growing bump!

Think of nutrition as a form of self-care, and an important one at that. What you eat makes an impression on your child, shaping everything from his or her brain development to taste preferences to metabolism. Proper nutrition also supports you and impacts your long-term health as you endure the demands of labor and breastfeeding. During this time when so many factors are beyond your control, take charge by eating right, engaging in physical activity that serves your body, and getting enough sleep. Any small changes you can make to improve your nutrition and overall health are worthwhile—perfection is overrated.

If you love science like we do, you will appreciate the research-based nutrition information in the following few pages. If you have a craving and need a delicious drink now, jump ahead to the recipes. You can come back to The Nutrition Primer when you are hungry for more information! In this chapter, we will take you on a whirlwind tour of nutrition during pregnancy, providing evidence-based guidance to empower you during this crucial time. This information is by no means comprehensive, so we provide a list of reputable resources in Appendix 5, Reliable Resources for Pregnancy, Nutrition, and Health (page 153), many of which informed the development of this chapter.

When it comes to nutrition, we keep an open mind, but we don't subscribe to fads and trends. Like you, we are constantly learning as the research rolls in and our field continues to evolve. Overall, we believe that labeling foods as "good" or "bad" is not the best practice, but there are some foods that should be limited and others that you can't go wrong eating—namely fruits and vegetables.

NUTRITION DURING PREGNANCY

Currently, the nutrition recommendations for pregnant women and those hoping to conceive are similar to those for the general population, with some additional considerations. Hopefully, as time goes on, more research will investigate women's health and pregnancy, and these guidelines will become more fine-tuned. That said, every woman's needs are different, both prior to, during, and after pregnancy. Thus, we can only provide general information based on the existing literature. It is important to work closely with your doctor and/or a dietitian to tailor goals to your specific needs, particularly if you have health conditions, allergies or intolerances, follow a vegetarian or vegan diet, or are carrying multiple children.

The recommended intake of many vitamins and minerals increases during pregnancy to accommodate the growth of your baby without sacrificing your needs. Thus, even a "perfect" diet—if that exists—can have gaps, particularly with respect to intake of certain vitamins and minerals. Several nutrients to pay close attention to are listed in Appendix 1, Important Nutrients (page 144), along with dietary sources. Talk to your doctor or dietitian about whether you should consider a prenatal multivitamin to ensure that you are meeting your needs. Keep in mind that supplements are not meant to compensate for a poor diet.

Universally, the best thing you can do is to eat nutrient-dense, rather than energy-dense, foods. What does this mean? Nutrient-dense foods are those that pack in a lot of nutritional value, namely vitamins and minerals, without a lot of calories. This translates to focusing on whole foods, or those that don't come with an ingredient label, while keeping added sugars, trans fats, and refined and highly processed foods to a minimum. Putting plant foods—fruits, vegetables, whole grains, legumes, and nuts—at the center of your diet will fill you with vitamins, minerals, fiber, and healthy fats to keep you at your best. That said, there should be some room for flexibility and to enjoy life!

Let's take a deeper dive into what a whole food diet approach means to us.

PLANT POWER

You may have heard the phrase "eat the rainbow," which conveys two important nutrition messages: choosing foods with vibrant, natural colors (fruits and vegetables) as well as eating a variety of plant foods. Fruits and vegetables are the foundation of any healthy dietary pattern at any stage of life. They are chock-full of vitamins and minerals (aka micronutrients) as well as phytochemicals, which not only give these foods their color and flavor but are a rich source of antioxidants. Be mindful that the skin is where you will find a lot of the nutritional value, so leave it on! In addition to micronutrients and phytochemicals, fruits and vegetables are an important source of fiber. Given the innumerable health benefits of consuming these foods, it was our top priority to develop drink recipes that incorporate whole fruits and even vegetables.

Whole grains, fruits, vegetables, and legumes are complex carbohydrates that are more slowly digested by the body due to the presence of fiber, which keeps your blood sugar from rising too high. These foods also retain vitamins and minerals that are lost during the refining process, for example, in making white flour and white rice. Beware! Many products are advertised as whole grain but may still include some refined flour, so be sure to double-check the ingredients label. Also, be mindful that "wheat flour" is different than whole wheat flour and may contain regular white flour as well.

All plants have some quantity of protein, with some packing in almost as much as animal foods. High protein foods include soy, legumes, nuts, seeds, and grains such as quinoa. Plant-based protein sources have the added benefit of containing healthy fats, micronutrients, and fiber. See Appendix 1, Important Nutrients (page 144) for more information on the importance of protein during pregnancy.

IS IT SAFE TO FOLLOW A VEGETARIAN OR VEGAN DIET DURING PREGNANCY?

According to the Academy of Nutrition and Dietetics, a vegetarian or vegan diet is "appropriate" for women who are pregnant or lactating but requires some extra planning. Several of the nutrients of concern for women who follow vegetarian or vegan diets include iron, vitamin B12, zinc, calcium, vitamin D, omega 3 fatty acids, and protein—many of these nutrients are the same as those that omnivorous mothers-to-be should be mindful of (see Appendix 1, Important Nutrients on page 144 for more information). Plant-based diets have numerous health benefits as well as positive implications for the environment and sustainability. Vegetarians and vegans typically have a lower Body Mass Index (BMI) and reduced risk for cardiovascular disease, diabetes, and cancer (particularly colon cancer). In the context of pregnancy, numerous studies have demonstrated that women who consumed plant-rich diets experienced fewer complications, including gestational diabetes and preeclampsia. In addition, children born to mothers consuming plant-rich diets exhibited healthy weight and length at birth. It is worth noting that the maternal diet patterns that were positively associated with desirable outcomes often included dairy, eggs, and fish: in other words, you do not have to go completely vegetarian or vegan to reap the benefits of a whole-food, plant-based diet!

ANIMAL PRODUCTS

Animal products have unique nutritional value, and we believe that you can incorporate these into a healthy dietary pattern in moderation—the name of the game is to choose wisely and be cautious of portion size. For example, when choosing meats and animals products, choose organic, grass-fed or pasture-raised. Always cook meat, fish, and eggs thoroughly to reduce the risk of foodborne illness (see our Appendix 2, Food Safety Considerations During Pregnancy on page 148 for more information). Fish is an excellent protein source for pregnant women and delivers essential fats (namely omega 3 fatty acids; see Appendix 1, page 147 for definition) that are important for your child's neurodevelopment and difficult to acquire from other food sources. While it is safe to consume fish during pregnancy (aim for 2-3 servings, for a total of 8-12 ounces per week), it is important to consider the type of fish (for example, choose low-mercury fish), sourcing, and preparation (see Appendix 2). Red and processed meats, including deli meats, hot dogs, bacon, sausage, and other smoked and cured meats, should be consumed in moderation, as high consumption has been linked to increased risk of death and chronic disease. For example, in a 2015 update to a previous report, the World Cancer Research Fund and American Institute for Cancer Research synthesized the literature on colon cancer, finding an increased risk with consumption of red and processed meats (12% for every 100 grams/day consumed).

Dairy offers protein, calcium, and fat-soluble vitamins (namely vitamins A and D). But should you choose full-fat, non-fat, or low-fat? The jury is out, but we believe that it depends on how your overall diet looks and that dairy in any form can be part of a balanced diet. The 2015-2020 Dietary Guidelines for Americans promotes low-fat dairy, which delivers fewer calories and less saturated fat, the type of fat that has been linked to cardiovascular disease and other chronic diseases. However, lower-fat dairy products are less satiating. In the case of yogurt and frozen products, more sugar may be added to improve flavor, which is arguably worse. In addition, there is evidence to suggest that one to two daily servings of whole milk dairy, namely yogurt, may be beneficial in the context of fertility. If you avoid dairy for any reason, there are lots of great milk and yogurt alternatives; including nut, soy, oat, and coconut. Like cow's milk, many non-dairy milks are fortified, meaning that vitamins and minerals are added to them. Each of the non-dairy milk options offers unique flavors, textures, and nutrient profiles: for example, hemp milk contains omega 3 fatty acids, and soy milk is high in protein relative to other non-dairy milks. There are even nut milks with added protein (usually pea protein). Regardless of which plant-based milk you choose, look for brands that are fortified to help meet your needs and opt for unsweetened versions to keep the added sugars to a minimum.

Eggs are an excellent source of protein, but if you throw away the yolk, you will miss out on some of the nutrition, including close to half of the protein content of the whole egg. In addition to protein, eggs offer fat-soluble vitamins (including vitamin A), essential fatty acids, and choline, all of which support the development of your baby, particularly his or her brain. Cholesterol from foods, like eggs, is less concerning to health professionals than it used to be. In fact, the 2015-2020 Dietary Guidelines for Americans did not include cholesterol as a nutrient for concern or place a suggested upper limit on consumption. A meta-analysis published in 2015 found that dietary cholesterol was not associated with increased risk of cardiovascular disease; though, the authors noted that more evidence is needed to clarify the relationship between cholesterol intake, blood lipids, and disease outcomes. Consuming eggs in moderation can support a healthy diet and pregnancy.

HOW MUCH SHOULD I EAT?

We have all heard the phrase "eating for two." As you may have realized, our book title was inspired by this common phrase. Instead of thinking about this as doubling how much you eat, focus on increasing the *quality* of your food choices to meet the needs of you and your baby. In fact, your energy (calorie) needs do not change in the first trimester, and then they increase by roughly 350 calories and 450 calories in the second and third trimesters, respectively. These values reflect what is needed to facilitate "normal" weight gain during the second and third trimesters but should be tailored to your pregnancy with guidance from your doctor and/or dietitian.

Most of us do not think of body fat in a positive way, but it is a hormonal organ that serves a purpose, especially during pregnancy. Having an optimal amount—not too much or too little—is essential to conception and carrying a pregnancy to term. It is also important for having adequate stored energy postpartum and for ensuring that hormones, including insulin, are in balance. With that said, many women are at risk for excessive weight gain, which has been linked with negative health effects for both mom and baby.

The desired trajectory of your weight gain depends on several factors: age, your normal weight, whether you have given birth previously, and your physical activity. According to the 2009 guidelines set forth by the Institute of Medicine, women within a "normal" range for weight prior to pregnancy should expect to gain 25-35 lbs during pregnancy. In addition to your growing bump, this weight manifests as increased breast tissue, increased maternal stores (for later stages of pregnancy and breastfeeding), and increased blood volume. Regardless of your circumstances, proper and well-managed weight gain is normal, and a critical aspect of having a healthy pregnancy and child. Your doctor will help you determine what is an appropriate amount and rate of weight gain. Particularly for women with a history of body image issues or disordered eating, the inevitability of weight gain may be difficult to accept, so seek help if this is something that you are struggling with.

FLUIDS

What you drink is just as important as what you eat! The Academy of Nutrition and Dietetics recommends that pregnant women consume three liters (roughly three quarts) of fluid per day. Some of this fluid may come from foods that have high water content, including fruits and vegetables, but most (around 10 cups) should be in the form of water or other nutritious beverages. As we will review in depth, it is best to keep caffeine and sugar-sweetened beverages, including soda, sports drinks, sweet tea, punch, and juice cocktails, to a minimum. Alcohol should be avoided completely.

ALCOHOL

Alcohol use and abuse is on the rise in the United States. A study published in 2017 revealed increases in the prevalence of alcohol use and high risk drinking behaviors among Americans (between 2001-2002 and 2012-2013). This was defined as four or more drinks in one occasion for women, and five or more for men. What's more, a 57.9% increase in high-risk drinking was observed in women, specifically.

The prevailing mentality is that a little bit of alcohol is fine, even beneficial, but heavy drinking increases risk of disease and mortality. However, recent evidence suggests that the current guidelines for alcohol consumption may be too lenient. Examining data from nearly 600,000 individuals from 19 high-income countries, researchers found that drinking more than five or six "standard" drinks per week (that is, more than 100 grams of alcohol) was associated with an increased risk of death due to any cause. For reference, the recommended upper limit in the U.S. is 196 grams of pure alcohol per week for men, or 14 standard drinks, and 98 grams, or seven standard drinks, for women. Wine was not found to be less harmful relative to beer or spirits.

1 STANDARD DRINK = 14 GRAMS PURE ALCOHOL
5 FLUID OUNCES OF WINE
12 FLUID OUNCES (1 CAN OR BOTTLE) BEER
1.5 FLUID OUNCES LIQUOR (1 SHOT)

In addition, alcohol intake has consistently been linked with breast cancer in women and other types of cancer in both men and women. For example, a 2015 analysis examining prospective data of women (and men) enrolled in the Health Professionals Study determined that consumption of up to one alcoholic drink per day (5-14.9 grams of pure alcohol a day) was associated with an increased risk of developing an alcohol-related cancer; this association was "driven" by breast cancer incidence. Again, drinking wine as opposed to other alcoholic beverages has not been found to be protective. Overall, we could all probably stand to be more moderate with our alcohol intake.

ALCOHOL AND PREGNANCY

If you picked up this book, you are probably trying to avoid alcoholic beverages during or in anticipation of pregnancy. According to a study published by the CDC in 2015, half of women of childbearing age consume alcohol, and 20% engaged in a binge drinking episode(s), defined as more than four drinks in one occasion, in the past 30 days. Why is this important? Because this study also reported that three in four women who wanted to get pregnant did not stop consuming alcohol prior to ditching their birth control methods. What's more, one in 10 pregnant women reported drinking within the past 30 days, with one in 33 reporting a binge drinking episode.

The effects of alcohol depend on the timing, dose, and pattern of exposure—but there is no known safe amount or stage of pregnancy to consume alcohol, a statement that is supported by the CDC, U.S. Surgeon General, and American Academy of Pediatrics. There is a misconception that a baby is less vulnerable to alcohol later in pregnancy, but the third trimester is the time when, among other things, the brain is undergoing a growth spurt, or a period of significant production of cells. Alcohol crosses the placenta unfiltered, and metabolism by the growing baby is much slower, allowing it to act for longer than it would in an adult human. Alcohol consumption during pregnancy increases the risk of mortality and can lead to birth defects and disabilities in the developing child. Collectively, the disorders that can result from alcohol exposure during pregnancy are called Fetal Alcohol Spectrum Disorders (FASD). These represent the leading preventable causes of developmental disorders in the United States. A study released in 2018 updated the statistics on prevalence of FASD's in the United States. Looking at four communities representing different regions, conservative estimates suggested that as many as 5% of first graders met the criteria for an FASD. While these results may not apply to all communities in the U.S., these statistics are still alarmingly high for something that is 100% preventable.

It is true that much of what we know about the negative effects of alcohol exposure come from animal studies, using models that may or may not be generalizable to humans. Researching the effects of alcohol in humans is very challenging for numerous reasons, including but not limited to ethics and stigmatization of women who admit to drinking while pregnant. Studies that have looked at light or moderate exposure to alcohol found mixed outcomes. In addition, some women anecdotally report having consumed alcohol while pregnant without consequence, and some doctors even tell their patients that one drink probably won't hurt. It is considered normal for women in other countries to drink while they are pregnant. But, in the words of a prominent alcohol researcher, when it comes to the controversy surrounding drinking while pregnant, the "absence of proof is not the proof of absence." Here's our two cents: with so much that could go wrong during a pregnancy that is out of your control, why take the risk with something that you can control?

In this section, we do not intend to scare anyone or to add any undue guilt or stress, but rather to inform and combat mixed messages. For pregnant women concerned about having consumed alcohol, consult your doctor. Start with a clean slate by taking better care of yourself today. For someone who is having a difficult time giving up alcohol or tobacco, consult a healthcare provider and seek help. One good resource is the Substance Abuse and Mental Health Services Administration National Hotline, with free, 24-hour assistance available to anyone. If you are planning to become pregnant or stop birth control methods, consider limiting or eliminating alcohol. Recent estimates suggest that about 50% of pregnancies are unplanned, and a woman may not know she is pregnant for several weeks.

A word on kombucha: when developing this book, we decided to refrain from making recipes with kombucha. This is due to the fact that kombucha contains alcohol. Typically, the level of alcohol is trace and below the threshold for being classified as an alcoholic beverage (0.5% alcohol by volume, or ABV). This is because the bacteria and yeast that make the bubbly 'booch work in harmony, with the yeast producing alcohol through fermentation and the bacteria gobbling it up and converting it to acid. However, if stored improperly or left for too long, the fermentation process can continue, producing more alcohol. In fact, in some instances, kombucha has been taken off the shelves, and there is an ongoing debate over whether to label kombucha as an alcoholic beverage. This prompted some brands to take action and start independently verifying the alcohol content of their kombucha. For brands that do not carry this "Verified Non-alcoholic" label, it may be difficult to know beyond a reasonable doubt how much alcohol is actually in these drinks when you pull them off the shelves. Furthermore, most kombuchas are raw, meaning not pasteurized (if they were, the process would kill all the probiotic value by eliminating the bacteria). Unpasteurized products of any kind are not recommended for pregnant women (see Appendix 2, Food Safety Considerations During Pregnancy on page 148 for more information). To avoid confusion, we avoided using kombucha in our recipes.

ADDED SUGARS

Added sugars are those that are not naturally found in foods, meaning they are added during processing. Foods with added sugars include the usual suspects—baked goods, candy, soda, ice cream—but also can be found in less obvious "healthy" foods like flavored yogurts (particularly those that are lower in fat), salad dressing, salsa and tomato sauce, granola, protein bars, and ready-to-eat cereals. Beverage products with added sugar include sports drinks, chocolate milk, punches, juice drinks (those that are not 100% fruit or vegetable), popular coffee and espresso drinks, and—the reason we're all here—cocktails. Looking for added sugars in food is not straightforward, as there are many names for these on food labels. See the box on the next page for names to look for on ingredient lists.

The 2015-2020 Dietary Guidelines for Americans recommends minimizing added sugars, limiting to less than 10% of energy intake. For someone consuming 2,000 calories a day, this is less than 200 calories from added sugars, or 50 grams per day—if you do the math, that is 12 teaspoons (one tsp = four grams sugar = 16 calories). As an example, a can of cola contains 40 grams of sugar, or 10 teaspoons.

Minimizing the intake of added sugars is important for several reasons. First, they are a source of extra calories that come without any nutritional value, also known as "empty calories." They either displace more nutrient-dense sources of energy or contribute to an increase in overall energy intake, which can lead to overeating and weight gain. In addition, both added sugars and refined grains have more extreme effects on blood glucose than do whole grains or fruits and vegetables that come with a fiber buffer. As we will discuss later in this chapter (see Complications – Gestational Diabetes, page 31), maintaining stable blood sugar levels during pregnancy is important to the normal growth and long-term health of your baby. Since cocktails and beverages are a source of hidden added sugar, it was important to us that we develop recipes that minimize and, for the most part, avoid the addition of sugar—even "natural" sugars.

COMMON NAMES FOR SUGAR

◆

anhydrous dextrose	honey	pancake syrup
brown sugar	invert sugar	raw sugar
confectioner's powdered sugar	lactose	sucrose
corn syrup	malt syrup	sugar
corn syrup solids	maltose	white granulated sugar
dextrose	maple syrup	
fructose	molasses	*Note that trending "natural" sweeteners, including maple syrup, honey, agave syrup, and coconut sugar, are still added sugar.*
high-fructose corn syrup (HFCS)	nectars (peach nectar, pear nectar)	

TO JUICE OR NOT TO JUICE?

Most Americans do not meet the recommended intakes for fruits and vegetables. 100% juice, namely fruit juice, is a convenient and inexpensive way for many Americans, including children, to meet their micronutrient requirements. It also offers antioxidants and other non-nutritive plant components, such as polyphenols, that may be beneficial for health. However, juice consumption is controversial because of its high sugar content and absence of fiber naturally present in whole fruits. In fact, the WHO classifies juice as a "free sugar," subject to a limit of less than 10% of total energy intake. In this sense, drinking juice could be, and is sometimes, compared to drinking soda.

There is much debate surrounding this topic, and research examining the effect of juice consumption on weight and other outcomes in adults and children is mixed; as with many areas in nutrition, the only consistent conclusion is that more research is needed. The current recommendations of the Dietary Guidelines for Americans are that adults should limit juice consumption of 100% juice to eight fluid ounces per day and instead focus on water and whole fruits. It is important to note, though, that juice cocktails and other juices with added sugars do not fall under this umbrella and should be limited.

We chose to include freshly-squeezed and 100% juices in our recipes, because we believe they serve a purpose, not the least of which is adding flavor and color to drinks. Most of our drink recipes include no more than a few ounces of juice, if any, and many are made with whole fruits. Like cocktails, our drinks should be consumed in moderation but can have a place in a healthy lifestyle and pregnancy. Unlike cocktails, we took measures to minimize or completely avoid adding sugar, syrup, and alternative sweeteners, to make our beverages a healthy swap. What's more, you are saving quite a few calories by removing the alcohol itself, seven calories per gram, in fact!

SUGAR SUBSTITUTES/ARTIFICIAL SWEETENERS/NON-NUTRITIVE SWEETENERS

Most sugar substitutes are Generally Recognized as Safe (GRAS) for consumption and are approved for use during pregnancy. The only exception is saccharin. Using sugar substitutes can help cut back on added sugars in the diet, but their use is somewhat controversial in terms of weight management. Some evidence suggests that chemical sweeteners may impact blood glucose levels by altering insulin release and the gut microbiome. In addition, a Canadian cohort study published in 2016 revealed that children born to women who consumed artificially sweetened beverages daily during pregnancy were up to two times more likely to be overweight at one year of age than children born to women who did not report drinking artificially sweetened beverages.

So, what about alternative sweeteners, like stevia? While these are also considered safe to consume, there is evidence to suggest that compounds found in some sweeteners, such as rebaudioside A which can be found in stevia products, can be transferred to breast milk—the health implications are not clear. In addition, taste buds adapt to very sweet tastes, so minimizing alternative sweeteners is advisable for developing a taste for a healthy diet. We refrained from using all artificial and non-nutritive sweeteners when developing our recipes.

CAFFEINE

Like many people, we love sipping a good cup (or two) o' joe to kick-start our mornings! But, similar to alcohol, caffeine is a drug that passes through the placenta to the baby, who is unable to process it like an adult. So, it is important to be mindful when consuming caffeinated beverages, including coffee, tea, and energy drinks. Other sources of caffeine to be aware of include some medications, including those for headaches, and chocolate. The literature on the impact of caffeine on the developing child is mixed, but the current recommendation is to limit your intake to 200 milligrams per day. This translates to 12 fluid ounces, or one and a half cups, of coffee a day; brewed teas have less caffeine. Consumption above this recommended threshold increases the risk of miscarriage among other complications. Be mindful that this is a rough estimate, as roasting and brewing impacts caffeine content of coffee. In addition, there is some evidence to suggest that caffeine intake may impact the weight and growth trajectory of the child. A recent study from Norway observed an association between caffeine consumption during pregnancy and having a child with a higher birth weight and a higher BMI at age eight; this relationship was strongest for high (more than 200mg/day) and very high caffeine intake (more than 300 mg/day).

A handful of our drinks are made with tea and coffee. Depending on how much caffeine you do (or don't) want to drink, feel free to use decaf brews or avoid these drinks altogether. Always consult your doctor about whether it is appropriate for you to continue to use caffeine.

SUPPLEMENTS, HERBS, AND TEAS

According to the Food and Drug Administration, a supplement contains "ingredients [such] as vitamins, minerals, herbs, amino acids, and enzymes. Dietary supplements are marketed in forms such as tablets, capsules, soft gels, gel caps, powders, and liquids." It is important to be aware that the onus is on manufacturing companies to ensure the quality (i.e. safety and effectiveness) of a supplement. The Food and Drug Administration (FDA) only reviews the safety of ingredients that they have not approved previously; thus, if all ingredients in a new supplement are considered safe by the FDA, the supplement can go to market without their oversight. It is also worth noting that the FDA does not verify health claims of supplements. Furthermore, the safety of many supplements, particularly herbal supplements, has not been evaluated in pregnant women. Be wary of promises that sound too good to be true. Always let your doctor know about any supplements that you are taking or plan to take.

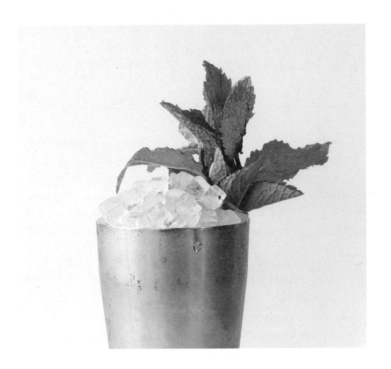

Herbal teas are non-caffeinated brews of components of plants, such as roots, flowers, and leaves—so they aren't actually "tea." Use caution when brewing herbal teas, as some contain ingredients that may not be safe for consumption during pregnancy, including those that are marketed to pregnant women. Ginger, peppermint, and chamomile teas are okay in moderation. For ginger and peppermint, try brewing your own tea by steeping fresh ginger or mint leaves. You can also steep fruit, peels, or spices to make your own decaf brews.

Red raspberry leaf tea is often promoted as being a "pregnancy tea," with purported benefits including diminishing menstrual cramps and preparing a woman's body to undergo childbirth. While these claims have not been validated scientifically, this herb is considered safe for consumption.

MANAGEMENT OF COMMON SYMPTOMS

So, now you know what you should be eating to achieve optimal nutrition for you and baby during pregnancy, but what if you don't feel like eating the "right" stuff? Common symptoms experienced during pregnancy might make you wonder whether you can meet these recommendations and how this might impact you and your baby. Here, we address common symptoms and strategies for managing them.

MORNING SICKNESS, NAUSEA, AND FOOD AVERSIONS

As many as 75% of women experience nausea and/or vomiting, much of which occurs early in the day—hence the name "morning sickness." Typically, this is confined to the first trimester, but the severity and duration can vary among women. A small percentage of women are affected by hyperemesis gravidarum, a condition marked by persistent, severe vomiting that contributes to weight loss and electrolyte imbalances that may require hospitalization. If you are concerned by your symptoms, speak to your doctor.

According to the Academy of Nutrition and Dietetics, the most common food aversions are to coffee, tea, fried or fatty foods, highly spiced foods, meat, and eggs. Often, these occur during the first trimester and may overlap with feelings of nausea. Nausea management during pregnancy is highly individualized and not well-studied, so it is helpful to keep track of your symptoms and triggers. Follow your instincts about what foods you feel like your body needs or can tolerate. Eat small meals or snacks throughout the day to avoid becoming too full or hungry. Anecdotal evidence suggests that ginger may help reduce nausea. We provide several drink recipes containing ginger as alternatives to ginger ale, the classic nausea beverage, but there are also chews and hard candies that could hit the spot. Carbonation may provide relief from nausea for some. Cold and room temperature foods and drinks may be less offensive. There is also limited evidence to suggest the benefit of vitamin B6. Food sources include banana, avocado, pineapple, spinach, chickpeas, and some nuts and seeds. Citrus may also work for some women.

When vomiting, it is important to focus on replacing fluids and electrolytes. Sip on water and beverages slowly throughout the day so as to not overload the stomach with fluid. Coconut water is great for replacing both lost fluids and electrolytes, and as such we use it in many of our recipes. Other foods high in potassium, including bananas, avocado, potato (regular and sweet), and winter squash are good options if tolerated.

CRAVINGS

Cravings—we all get them. They can result from learned associations, often emotional or even nostalgic, like chocolate makes us happy and mac & cheese brings us comfort. They can also tell us when we might be lacking certain nutrients. Normal hormonal fluctuations that occur during menstruation and pregnancy are partly to blame, as they can suppress our feelings of fullness and drive us to reach for foods with lower nutritional value. Common food cravings during pregnancy include chocolate, citrus fruits, pickles, chips, and ice cream. Cravings for sweets tend to peak mid-gestation. Managing cravings in a healthy and balanced way is an art and a science, and we hope that our recipes provide you with nutritious options for when you get a hankering. If you are chewing on ice or experiencing non-food cravings, such as cornstarch or baking soda, let your physician know, as these can be indicative of more severe nutrient deficiencies.

TASTE AND SMELL CHANGES

Some women experience changes to their sense of taste and smell, making them more sensitive to strong smells and flavors. Avoid strong smells and flavors, such as spicy foods—again, go with your gut, pun intended. Adding acid (from citrus, for example) to foods can reduce metallic tastes. Chewing gum may also help. Having someone else prepare food or drinks for you may also be helpful with sensitivities to smells.

CONSTIPATION

It's true, doctors and dietitians love talking about poop—because it can tell you a lot about what is going on inside your body! Changes in digestion are a normal part of pregnancy resulting from hormonal fluctuations in the body, changes to the organization of the abdominal cavity, decreased physical activity, and even supplementation (namely with iron). To manage constipation, make sure that you are drinking enough water and achieving an optimal intake of fiber—not too much or too little—by focusing on eating fruits, vegetables, whole grains, and legumes. If you are working to improve your diet by increasing your intake of fiber-rich foods, do so slowly and ensure that you are likewise increasing your intake of water. Finally, exercise can help keep things moving, so consult your physician about what level of physical activity is appropriate for you.

REFLUX

Many women experience acid reflux, more commonly known as heartburn. This can happen at any time during pregnancy but is more common during the third trimester. Many of the previous recommendations will also help with management of this condition: eating small, frequent meals, drinking fluids and getting enough fiber to keep things moving; and avoiding high-fat, spicy, and other irritating foods. For women with reflux, citrus and carbonation may exacerbate symptoms. Mint may also be irritating.

SWELLING

Swelling is a normal pregnancy symptom. However, sudden changes in fluid may be indicative of something more serious. As always, check with your doctor if you have concerns. Prevent accumulation of fluid in your lower body by avoiding standing or sitting for extended periods of time. Elevate your feet above the level of your heart when at rest and wear loose fitting clothes. In terms of nutrition, make sure that you are achieving the right balance of fluid and sodium. Getting enough potassium is also important, as it acts as the counterpart to sodium and is essential to normal kidney function. Most fruits and veggies offer potassium, but sources with a higher potassium to sodium ratio include bananas, oranges and orange juice, avocados, prune juice, raisins, potatoes, and coconut water.

COMPLICATIONS

Gestational diabetes (GDM), or insulin resistance during pregnancy, poses risks to the developing child as well as the mother and may impact as many as 18% of pregnancies. Some degree of insulin resistance is actually normal and is the result of a storm of placental hormones and increased adipose tissue, typically beginning in the second half of pregnancy. These changes serve a purpose—to enable more glucose in your blood to be delivered to your baby, who needs it for fuel as it develops rapidly. However, for some women, the pancreas, which is the organ that makes insulin, cannot meet the demand for insulin production, leading to higher than desired blood glucose levels, or hyperglycemia. Your child, in turn, must increase his or her insulin production to manage incoming glucose, which may impact your child's weight and insulin resistance down the line. Along these lines, gestational diabetes has been linked to macrosomia, or high birth weight of the child, and other complications during pregnancy or delivery. Though GDM often resolves after birth, women who develop GDM have a higher risk—35-60%—of developing Type II diabetes within the next 10-20 years. Among other factors, carrying extra weight going into pregnancy increases the risk of developing GDM.

Preeclampsia affects 3-5% of pregnancies and is a serious condition that is dangerous for both mom and baby. Preeclampsia is characterized by high blood pressure (hypertension), which your doctor should monitor continuously, and protein in the urine. The recommendations for a healthy pregnancy, such as eating well and exercising moderately, will help prevent this complication.

PRECONCEPTION NUTRITION

Being as healthy as possible prior to pregnancy will give you the best shot at conceiving and having a healthy pregnancy. This includes managing your weight and any pre-existing conditions, such as prediabetes or diabetes. Evidence suggests that moderate weight loss (5-10%) in overweight women may improve fertility and reduce the risk of pregnancy-related complications. In their book, *The Fertility Diet*, Harvard researchers Jorge Chavarro, Walter Willett, and Patrick Skerrett recommend aiming for the sweet spot of 7.5% weight loss. A prospective study in Canada examining the relationship between pre-pregnancy BMI and maternal and infant outcomes suggests that women whose BMI's differ by 10% have "clinically meaningful risk differences" of experiencing complications. Always talk to your doctor or dietitian about whether weight loss is appropriate for you and your body in the context of your medical history and current health.

A healthy eating pattern prior to pregnancy that focuses on whole foods and incorporates a variety of plant foods will help you meet

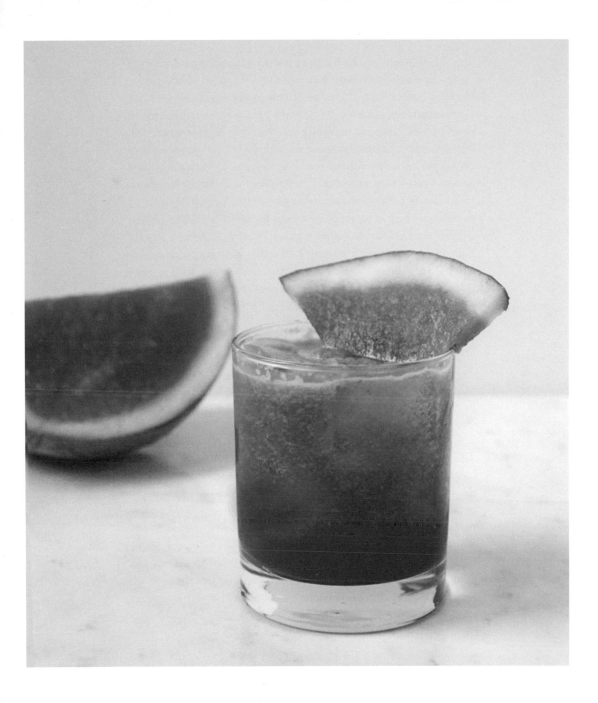

your micronutrient needs. Many vitamins and minerals are essential to development, particularly during the earliest stages of pregnancy, including, but not limited to, folate. This is particularly important, since many women may not know for sure whether they are pregnant for up to several weeks after conception. If you are trying to get pregnant, talk with your doctor or dietitian about any blood work that may shed light on your current nutrient status, how to optimize your diet in the context of dietary restrictions, and whether supplementation may be beneficial.

Moderate caffeine and alcohol consumption prior to pregnancy, to date, has not been associated with impaired fertility; however, either in excess likely has negative effects. This appears to be true for both men and women. It is worth noting that designing high-quality studies to test these research questions is challenging, and, as mentioned in the book *The Fertility Diet*, alcohol in particular certainly will not help you get pregnant.

POSTPARTUM NUTRITION

◆

The postpartum period is extremely important for both mom and baby, and thus is often referred to as the "fourth trimester." Though the focus of this section is nutrition after birth, we want to take the opportunity to impress upon new moms and moms-to-be the importance of monitoring *your* health after birth, taking seriously any abnormal symptoms that arise, and working closely with your doctor to develop a postpartum care plan. Currently, in the U.S., as many as 50,000 women a year experience severe maternal morbidity, which refers to any "unexpected outcomes of labor and delivery that result in significant short- or long-term consequences to a woman's health."

These complications include preeclampsia, infection from tears or placental remnants, and blood clots, among others. The rate of death and near-death experiences after childbirth is much higher in the U.S. relative to other developed countries; in fact, an American woman has three times the risk of dying relative to a woman from Canada or Britain. Fortunately, the importance of maternal health is being better recognized. In May 2018, the American College of Obstetricians & Gynecologists released a Committee Opinion recommending that observation and care of women postpartum be "ongoing" rather than limited to a single visit six weeks after birth. This information is not meant to scare anyone, but rather to inform and to encourage new mothers to be their own health advocates. Talk with your doctor about what you should expect after delivery and what symptoms might be cause for concern.

Postpartum nutrition is important, as you are not only replenishing your own stores and facilitating your post-birth recovery, but you may also be the sole source of nutrition for another human being if you choose to breastfeed. Breast milk is generally considered to be the best, most complete source of nutrition for a child, and breastfeeding provides many short- and long-term benefits to the mom and baby. The American Academy of Pediatrics recommends exclusive breastfeeding for the first six months of life. However, whether to breastfeed or not is a personal choice and may not be the best option for all mother-infant pairs. Talk with your doctor about what is appropriate for you and your baby, and don't be afraid to seek help from your physician or a lactation specialist if you are struggling with breastfeeding. Breastfeeding moms require additional energy, about 300-400 additional calories depending on the stage. What you eat affects the composition of breast milk, which in turn determines the nutrients that your baby receives. Among other nutrients of concern, it is important to get enough DHA, an essential fatty acid that is crucial for brain and eye development and can be found in fish and eggs; a supplement may be indicated if you do not consume these foods.

Many women are concerned with losing weight after pregnancy, but there is no rush. Eating a balanced diet as previously described and engaging in physical activity per the direction of your doctor will facilitate gradual, healthy weight loss. One of the benefits of breastfeeding is that it helps mothers return to pre-pregnancy weight, in combination with a diet that meets (but does not exceed) enhanced energy needs. Cutting calories, particularly while breastfeeding, is not recommended, and eating less than 1,800 calories per day may negatively impact your ability to properly nourish your baby through breastfeeding.

With that said, aiming to return to pre-pregnancy weight is often important for long-term health. For example, obese women who lost weight between pregnancies (for reference, as little as 12 pounds for a woman 5ft. 4in.) significantly reduced the risk of having a baby with a higher than desired birth weight at their subsequent pregnancy. Weight loss between pregnancies also reduces the risk of developing gestational diabetes and preeclampsia.

Women who are breastfeeding may choose to consume an occasional alcoholic beverage but should allow at least two to three hours before pumping or breastfeeding to allow the body sufficient time to metabolize the alcohol. Remember, the greater the amount of alcohol consumed on an occasion, the higher the blood alcohol concentration and the longer it takes to metabolize and clear the alcohol from one's system. Alcohol does get into breastmilk and thus can be transferred to your baby. In addition, it can impact hormones, such as oxytocin, related to lactation, impairing your ability to breastfeed while it is active in your system.

LET'S HEAR IT
FOR THE MEN!

◆

Research investigating the importance of paternal nutrition is growing, but much of the existing knowledge comes from animal studies. For example, higher weight and poor diet quality have both been associated with decreased sperm motility, increased risk of sperm abnormality, including alterations to the genetic material, and hormonal imbalances in males: for example, lower testosterone and increased estradiol. Rodent studies have demonstrated that offspring of male animals fed a poor diet experienced negative effects, such as insulin resistance and increased weight. As with female fertility, it is unclear whether caffeine and alcohol impact male fertility.

HOW DOES THIS BOOK
FIT INTO EVERYTHING WE
JUST TALKED ABOUT?

◆

We hope that by giving you a taste of the importance of healthy eating (and drinking!) before, during, and after pregnancy, we have provided you with some clarity and empowered you to take control of your health today, starting with what goes in your glass. All of our mocktail recipes are booze-free, low in added sugar, and made with nutritious ingredients that are safe for pregnancy but appropriate for anyone.

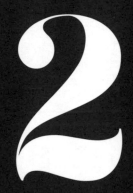

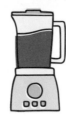

MAKING A
MOCKTAIL

◆

I n this chapter, we will help you get your kitchen set up so that you can
make any of our drinks whenever the mood strikes! Here, we review
the kitchen appliances, tools, and glassware you'll need, teach you a few
basic bartending techniques, and highlight a number of ingredients to
have on hand.

In addition to avoiding excess sugar, we want to avoid adding any
stress to your routine with our drink recipes. We hope you'll find that our
mocktails are easier to prepare than you might think—no prior bartending
experience required! Most of our recipes only take a few minutes to throw
together using ingredients, methods, and tools that are widely available.
All of our recipes make two servings, except the batch recipes which are
meant to serve larger groups.

TOOLS OF THE TRADE

———————————◆———————————

Proper tools are essential to making any recipe a reality. Our mock-tails are no exception. The good news is that you may have most of these tools and appliances in your kitchen already! If not, and you prefer not to purchase anything, we provide suggestions and alternatives when we can.

HIGH-POWER BLENDER

A high-power blender is necessary to prepare many of our mocktails, namely those that are frozen. For smaller quantities or softer ingredients, a food processor works fine, too.

SHAKER

A shaker helps to mix and cool ingredients with the addition of ice and serves as a great holder for muddling. There are two types of shakers, a cobbler shaker and a Boston shaker. A cobbler shaker, commonly referred to as a three-piece cocktail shaker, has a built-in strainer and is more often used by beginners. A Boston shaker comes with a Boston glass (also known as a metal tumbler) and a separate strainer, either a hawthorne or julep strainer. The Boston shaker is often favored by bartenders, because it holds more volume, making it more efficient when dealing with a busy crowd. Either one works for this book. If you don't want to purchase a shaker, feel free to improvise. Find a shaker lid for a mason jar, use a travel coffee mug, or as a last resort, reach for a reusable water bottle—all of which were used at some point by us in the making of these recipes!

FINE MESH STRAINER, CHEESECLOTH, OR NUT MILK BAG

We like to offer you the option of "pulp or no pulp" in a few of our drinks. A fine mesh strainer, cheesecloth, or a nut milk bag can be used interchangeably to strain out any undesired ingredient bits. Don't have any of these on hand? Then, keep the pulp! Your drink will still taste great and include a nutritional boost.

MUDDLER

Muddling is a technique we use frequently throughout the book, as it helps bring out the flavor of fresh fruit and herbs. A muddler is a long bar tool with an enlarged tip, usually made of wood or steel. Either type of muddler works for our recipes. You can find muddlers online or purchase one wherever you normally buy basic kitchen tools. If purchasing a muddler is not an option, you can use the back of a mixing/baking spoon or whisk instead. We did this with a handful of recipes.

CITRUS JUICER

We recommend that you purchase a citrus juicer. Many of our recipes call for freshly squeezed lemon, lime, or orange juice, to name a few. You can order a basic citrus juicer online for as little as seven dollars or pick one up anywhere that stocks basic kitchen tools. Prefer not to buy a citrus juicer? Put those hands to work and squeeze!

REUSABLE OR RECYCLABLE STRAWS

Not a must-have, but straws are a fun addition to mocktails and can make some drinks, like our frozen ones, easier to sip. To be environmentally friendly, we suggest purchasing bamboo, paper, or metal straws.

BASIC TECHNIQUES

◆

We're nutrition professionals, not mixologists, and had no bartending experience prior to creating these recipes. Here are some basic techniques we learned along the way, and if we can learn them, trust us, so can you. Instead of repeating them with each recipe, we summarized the tricks of the trade in this "How To" section.

HOW TO USE A SHAKER

- ◆ Pour your ingredients into the shaker or glass and fill halfway with ice, unless indicated otherwise. Note that some recipes call for "dry shaking," which means shaking ingredients without the addition of ice.

- ◆ Depending on what shaker you are using, place the lid or metal tumbler on securely.

- ◆ For the Boston shaker, make sure that the top metal tumbler is well sealed to the bottom glass by tapping the bottom of the tumbler with the heel of your hand.

- ◆ Using both hands (for the Boston shaker, place one hand on the glass and one on the tumbler), shake vigorously over your shoulder for at least 10 slow-counting seconds.

- ◆ Strain the mixture into glasses.

- ◆ For the cobbler shaker, you will be able to strain through the top piece of the shaker. For the Boston shaker, you will use a separate strainer. To break the seal between the top and bottom glasses before straining, use the heel of your hand to carefully but assertively tap the rim of the glass. This may take a few tries.

HOW TO MUDDLE

◆ Place herbs and/or fruit at the bottom of a glass or shaker.

◆ Using a muddler, gently press down on the herbs and/or fruit and twist three or four times.

◆ The goal is to slightly bruise the herbs but not break them; a good way to measure this is through smell. For example, if it starts to smell minty, you're in good shape!

HOW TO RIM A GLASS

Rims are often an essential part of the experience of drinking a cocktail, and we encourage you to follow the recipe if it calls for rimming. Rimming a glass is a great way to add to and complement existing flavors—hello, salted margaritas!

◆ Dry ingredients are the ingredients placed on the rim. In this book, you'll see salt for margaritas and crushed nuts or graham crackers for various dessert drinks. Use a plate or shallow bowl to hold your dry ingredients.

◆ Wet ingredients are used to stick the dry ingredients to the rim. We use several methods to wet the rim of a glass. These include sliding a lime wedge or piece of fruit around the rim or pouring a liquid like maple syrup in a plate or shallow bowl then dipping the rim. You can also use your fingers by dipping them into the liquid and sliding them around the glass.

◆ Lastly, dip and twist. After wetting the rim of the glass, turn the glass upside down and dip into your dry mixture. Gently twist the glass. Repeat until the rim is covered with the desired amount of dry ingredients.

INGREDIENTS TO HAVE ON HAND

In this section, we provide you with a list of basic ingredients to have on hand so when the urge to make a mocktail hits, you'll be ready! We avoided creating recipes with obscure, hard-to-find ingredients. Instead, we use ones you can easily purchase at your local supermarket or convenience store. Bonus: many of the ingredients can be used for multiple recipes.

We also took this opportunity to explain some key differences in ingredients that may slightly change the taste of a drink, like club soda vs. seltzer water. The good news is that our recipes are easily adapted, so feel free to get creative and branch out. With that said, we can't guarantee the same "results" (in taste or look) if you depart from the written recipes. We spent a lot of time testing and trying different ingredients, methods, and quantities, and what we provided in this book are the fruits of our efforts. And if you're like us and detest wasting leftover ingredients, do not worry! We provide you with tips and ideas for how to use extra ingredients throughout the book.

SPARKLING MINERAL WATER VS. SELTZER VS. CLUB SODA

The first section of our book is entitled, "Bubbly Drinks," which are nothing more than drinks made with carbonated water. In addition to providing a fun mouthfeel and enhancing taste, the carbonation may provide relief from nausea.

There are three basic types of carbonated water: sparkling mineral water, seltzer, and club soda. Sparkling mineral water is naturally carbonated water, usually from a spring or well, with naturally occurring minerals like salts and sulfur compounds. Seltzer is plain water that has been artificially carbonated. Because it's artificially carbonated, the bubbly sensation tends to be stronger than sparkling mineral water, and it's usually much cheaper. Lastly, club soda is carbonated water with the addition of minerals. These minerals, potassium sulfate, sodium chloride, and sodium bicarbonate to name a few, slightly change the taste of the carbonated water, often giving it a slightly saltier taste. The type and quantity of minerals added to club soda depend on the manufacturer. As you have probably experienced, leaving any type of carbonated water open for an extended period of time will contribute to its flatness, causing drinks to taste watered down; always use fresh carbonated water for drinks. We recommend seltzer for our recipes as it's 1) typically cheaper than its alternatives, 2) strongly carbonated, and 3) contains no artificial minerals. However, feel free to taste each one and decide which you prefer for your beverages. Just be sure to buy it plain, with no added flavors or sweeteners.

COCONUT WATER

Coconut water is used in many of our recipes. For those dealing with morning sickness, coconut water can help replenish fluids and electrolytes lost with vomiting. Plus, coconut water adds a touch of natural sweetness. Any brand is fine, but look for one that is pasteurized and contains no added sugar. The best way to avoid added sugar is to make sure it's not listed in the ingredients.

JUICE

We encourage squeezing your own juice as much as possible in our recipes; however, we figured we'd save you the hassle of juicing some fruit (ahem, pomegranates). When squeezing fresh juice, wash and dry the fruits well before cutting into them, and use them immediately. If purchasing juice, always avoid unpasteurized juice (see Appendix 2, Food Safety Considerations During Pregnancy on page

148), and when possible, opt for 100% juice with no added sugar. Citrus juice, namely from lemons and limes, is a staple ingredient used throughout our book, enhancing the flavors and adding tartness and sweetness to our beverages. We recommend freshly squeezed juice over bottled, as it's more flavorful and free of preservatives.

Throughout the book, we tell you how many tablespoons or cups of citrus juice to add to a drink. Below, we provide a reference for how much fruit you need to squeeze to get that amount of juice. This will vary with the size and ripeness of your fruit, but hopefully it will give you a sense of how much of these fruits to have on hand!

- **LEMON**
  1 lemon = 2 tbsp juice

- **LIME**
  1 lime = 2 tbsp juice

- **ORANGE**
  1 orange = ¼ cup juice

- **GRAPEFRUIT**
  1 grapefruit =
  ½ cup juice

GINGER

Ginger has been used as a natural remedy for nausea and vomiting for centuries. Plus, it provides a spicy, zesty flavor to our drinks. We offer several recipes containing ginger as an alternative to ginger ale. You may notice our recipes may say "1 tsp peeled and chopped ginger." This simply means peel the outer skin off the ginger using a peeler or paring knife, chop it into pieces, and then measure in a teaspoon. Depending on how well your blender works, the ginger may or may not blend into small, unnoticeable pieces. You can always strain out any large pieces or, better yet, chew or swallow them for extra nausea relief and a nutritional boost. Ginger can stay fresh for about a week at room temperature, and close to a month in the refrigerator. Of note, ground ginger has a much more concentrated flavor than fresh ginger and will not work well as a replacement in the recipes.

FRESH HERBS

Fresh herbs, such as mint, basil, and thyme, are used in many of our recipes. Herbs offer a range of nutritional benefits and add wonderful flavor to drinks. Unfortunately, herbs tend to go bad rather quickly, so it's best to buy them when you plan on making a mocktail. If you've bought herbs before, you may have experienced tossing a decent amount away. To avoid this, we provide you with fun tips and recipe ideas for any extra herbs.

NON-DAIRY MILK

You'll see "non-dairy milk" in a handful of our recipes. Feel free to use your favorite: almond, oat, coconut, soy, etc. Most non-dairy milks can be used interchangeably in these recipes unless stated otherwise (for example, we recommend coconut milk for the Piña Col-nada, page 99). We also recommend buying unsweetened, unflavored non-dairy milks (as opposed to those flavored with vanilla) and adding non-alcoholic vanilla extract when it is called for, as this will create a stronger, tastier flavor. If you prefer to use cow's milk to make drinks, be sure to purchase pasteurized and avoid "raw" milk (see Appendix 2, Food Safety Considerations During Pregnancy on page 148).

COCONUT MILK

Coconut milk comes in many different varieties including in a car-ton, in a can, regular, and lite. What's the difference? To put it simply, water content. Varying amounts of water are added to coconut cream to lighten it to different extents.

When you head down the ethnic foods aisle in your local grocery store, you may come across canned coconut milk. Some cultures use canned coconut milk in traditional recipes, such as coconut rice and curries. We use this kind of coconut milk to add a creamy texture to some of our drinks including our Pumpkin Pie Mock-tini (page 110), White-ish Russian (page 91), and Mocha-nut (page 100). We chose the regular kind as opposed to the lite version for taste and texture purposes, but feel free to switch to lite if you want to decrease the fat and calories.

When you head to the dairy aisle, you may notice coconut milk in a carton (similar to almond milk). This is essentially canned coconut milk watered down to the greatest extent. In our recipes, we always indicate which type of coconut milk to use, either coconut milk (canned) or coconut milk (carton) to help you avoid confusion. When coconut milk (canned) sits out for a while, the contents may separate. We recommend either giving it a good shake or blending it up in a food processor before using. If you select coconut milk as your "non-dairy milk" of choice, go for the carton version.

FRESH OR FROZEN FRUIT

As we mentioned, it was imperative for us to develop drink recipes that incorporate whole fruits whenever possible as a way to preserve the nutritional content, namely fiber. You'll see a range of fruits including berries, bananas, avocados, and dates in our recipes. We often give you the option to use fresh or frozen fruit. Frozen fruit has the same nutritional value as fresh fruit, and you don't have to worry about it going bad. Keep frozen blueberries, strawberries, mango, and pineapple on hand. You can even peel, slice up, and freeze ripe bananas for later use. Always wash fresh produce well before consuming.

DATES

You may notice dates in a few of our recipes. Dates are a naturally sweet fruit packed with lots of nutrients. Dates provide antioxidants, fiber, and vitamins like potassium and B6. When there's opportunity to blend a drink, we chose dates as our sweetener, so you can reap the benefits of their nutritional content while enjoying their sweetness. We prefer medjool dates, but other dates will work fine. In the directions, we recommend soaking dates. While this is optional, soaking the dates in water for about 10 minutes helps to soften them up and facilitates blending.

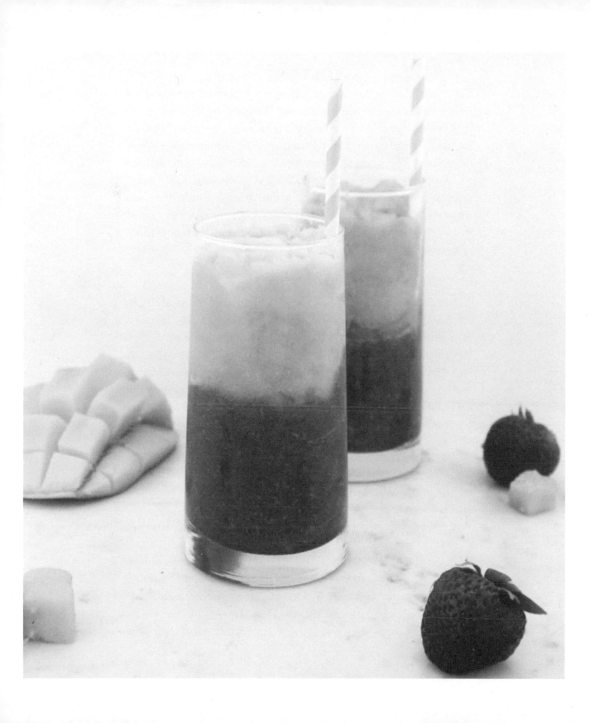

SWEETENERS

For a handful of recipes, we needed to add a touch of sweetness but couldn't use dates for various reasons: for example, the drink didn't require blending, the dates changed the flavor too much, etc. Instead, we used a small amount of light agave syrup, honey, maple syrup, or molasses. We keep the quantities to a minimum, but feel free to adjust the sweetness according to your preference. Light agave syrup or honey can be used interchangeably while maple syrup and molasses are purposely used in other drinks to complement certain flavor combinations. When choosing honey, look for pasteurized, not raw, honey.

APPLE CIDER VINEGAR

Yes, we use apple cider vinegar in our drinks! Before you entirely brush off this ingredient, hear us out. Apple cider vinegar may help with acid reflux, and we found it adds a "bite" similar to that of alcohol. We use minimal amounts, so don't worry about it being overpowering. And if you're experiencing heightened senses from pregnancy, feel free to reduce the quantities. Be sure to buy filtered, pasteurized apple cider vinegar (see Appendix 2, Food Safety Considerations During Pregnancy on page 148).

GLASSWARE

We created our drinks with the "standard" glassware listed in the table on the next page in mind. That is, our Chocolate Cream Martini is made to fit a standard martini glass, our Ging-osa and Belly-ni are suited for champagnes glasses, our Pine-alapeño Mojito is best served in a highball glass, and so on. As previously mentioned, each recipe, apart from the batch ones, is intended to make two servings. If your drinks don't quite fill the glasses up to the brim, it may be because you're using a slightly larger glass than the average-sized glass. We tried to stick with standard amounts for drinks as much as possible to not only give you the real feel of having an alcoholic drink but also to keep portion sizes in check—these drinks are healthier than their counterparts, but the calories will still add up! Below we provide you with references for estimated pours for each drink. Note, we also factored ice into how much volume a drink makes.

GLASSES

◆

AMOUNT OF FLUID OUNCES

SHOTS.. 1.5 OZ

MARTINI... 4-6 OZ

LOWBALL GLASS................................. 4-6 OZ

WINE & CHAMPAGNE........................ 4-5 OZ

HIGHBALL GLASS................................8-10 OZ

MUG.. 8-12 OZ

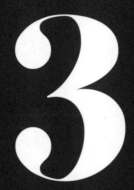

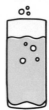

BUBBLY
DRINKS

M any of the drinks in this category are ideal for the first trimester, which is when you might experience nausea or morning sickness. These concoctions are carbonated, light in flavor, and made with classic nausea remedies, such as mint (see Mock-jito and variations), ginger (see Mock Mules and variations), and citrus juice. Cider vinegar may also be good for settling a turbulent tummy. Finally, coconut water not only adds a hint of natural sweetness to drinks but also replenishes electrolytes lost when vomiting.

MOCK-JITO

HIGHLIGHTS & BENEFITS
Hydrating ◆ May relieve nausea

This twist on the classic Cuban cocktail is refreshing and light, perfect on a hot day. Our formulation has just enough sweetness to balance the tartness of the lime juice and brighten the flavor of the fresh mint.

SERVES 2

INGREDIENTS
20 mint leaves

2 lime wedges

2 tsp light agave syrup

1 tsp apple cider vinegar

⅔ cup coconut water

¾–1 cup seltzer

2 cups ice

Additional mint leaves for garnish

TOOLS
Muddler

Citrus Juicer

Shaker

PREPARATION

1. Muddle mint leaves and lime wedges with the agave syrup and apple cider vinegar in the bottom of the shaker.

Don't throw away the muddled mint or extra mint from your drink. Instead, use it to make a second round (though the flavor may be slightly diluted).

2. Add coconut water and ice. Shake vigorously.

3. Fill glasses with ice and divide the shaken mixture, including the muddled mint and lime wedges, between the two glasses.

4. Top with seltzer and stir.

5. Garnish with mint sprigs.

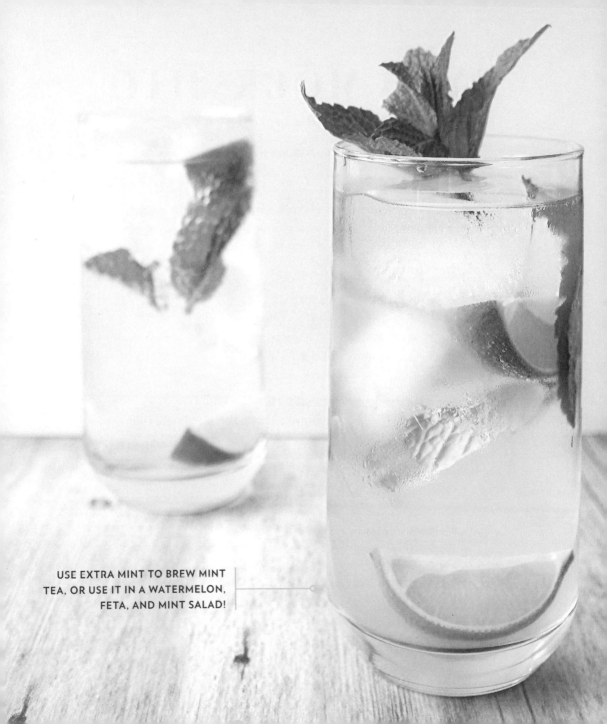

USE EXTRA MINT TO BREW MINT
TEA, OR USE IT IN A WATERMELON,
FETA, AND MINT SALAD!

BYOB MOCK-JITO

(BUILD YOUR OWN BERRY)

HIGHLIGHTS & BENEFITS

Contains antioxidants • Hydrating • May relieve nausea • No added sugar

Although sugar is an ingredient in many cocktails, here we use nature's sweetener—fruit! This drink would be great for a gender reveal or baby shower since you can use blue or pink berries!

SERVES 2

INGREDIENTS

20 fresh mint leaves

2 lime wedges

2 cups fresh or frozen berries, plus more for garnish (thaw if frozen)

We tested with raspberries and blueberries, but blackberries and strawberries will work too!

1 tsp apple cider vinegar

1 tsp lime juice

⅔ cup coconut water

½–¾ cup seltzer

2 cups ice

Additional mint leaves and berries for garnish

Optional: 1–2 tsp light agave

TOOLS

Blender or food processor

Citrus Juicer

Muddler

Shaker

PREPARATION

1. To make berry puree: blend berries with coconut water, apple cider vinegar, and lime juice.

2. Muddle the lime wedges and mint leaves in a shaker.

3. Add ice and berry puree to shaker. Shake vigorously.

4. Fill glasses with ice and divide the shaken mixture, including the muddled mint and lime wedges, between the two glasses.

5. Top with seltzer and stir.

6. Garnish with mint sprigs and berries.

TOSS LEFTOVER BERRIES IN A SALAD OR FREEZE THEM TO USE IN A SORBET.

MINTY-GREEN MOCK-JITO

HIGHLIGHTS & BENEFITS
Hydrating • Provides a boost of folate

Get your folate and iron-rich greens with this mojito! We love the vibrant color of this beverage, and it's so nutritious, you can even drink it for breakfast!

SERVES 2

INGREDIENTS

1–2 cups baby spinach or kale

Kale will taste more bitter, so you may need to up the sweetness.

1 medium apple

Choose a sweet variety, like Pink Lady or Honeycrisp. Pear would also be nice!

2 tbsp lime juice

1 orange, peeled

20 mint leaves

1 cup seltzer

2 cups ice

Optional: ¼ cucumber

Optional: blend in a date for added sweetness

TOOLS

Juicer or blender

Citrus Juicer

Strainer

PREPARATION

1. Muddle the mint leaves in the bottom of two highball glasses.

2. Prepare juice by running all ingredients (except seltzer and ice) through a juicer.

If you don't have a juicer, blend and then strain through cheesecloth. You will likely need to add liquid (we recommend 1 cup of coconut water), but this technique works really well!

3. Top with seltzer and ice; stir.

USE YOUR OWN GREEN JUICE OR PURCHASE A PASTEURIZED VERSION. THIS WOULD ALSO MAKE A GREAT MOJITO SMOOTHIE, A GOOD WAY TO KEEP ALL OF THE FRUIT AND VEGETABLE FIBERS.

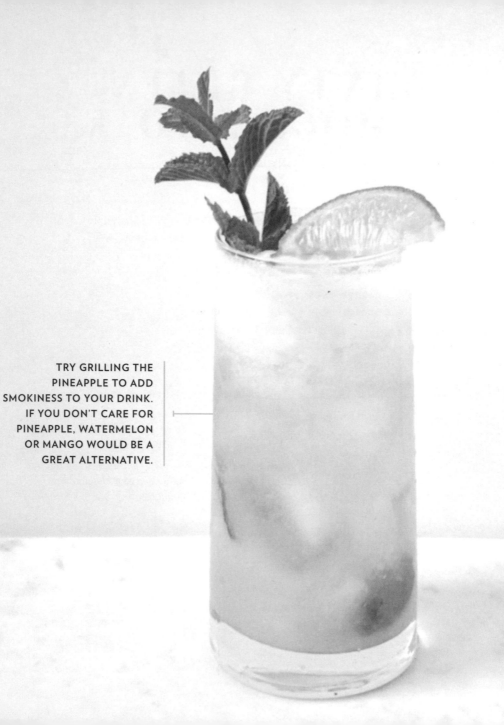

TRY GRILLING THE
PINEAPPLE TO ADD
SMOKINESS TO YOUR DRINK.
IF YOU DON'T CARE FOR
PINEAPPLE, WATERMELON
OR MANGO WOULD BE A
GREAT ALTERNATIVE.

PINE-JALAPEÑO MOCK-JITO

HIGHLIGHTS & BENEFITS
Anti-inflammatory • Made with whole fruit

If you're into sweet heat, this is the drink for you! Pineapples are rich in an enzyme called bromelain, which may help reduce inflammation, swelling, and even bruising.

SERVES 2

INGREDIENTS

20 fresh mint leaves

2 lime wedges

2 cups diced fresh or frozen pineapple (thaw if frozen)

2-4 thinly sliced rounds of jalapeño or as desired, seeds removed

The amount of jalapeño you use will depend on the heat of your pepper and your tolerance. Remove seeds for mild heat; leave seeds for more intense heat.

1 tsp apple cider vinegar

1 tsp lime juice

⅔ cup coconut water

½-¾ cup seltzer

2 cups ice

Additional mint leaves, pineapple, and jalapeño slices for garnish

Optional: 1-2 tsp light agave

TOOLS

Blender or food processor

Citrus Juicer

Muddler

Shaker

PREPARATION

1. To make pineapple puree: blend pineapple with coconut water, lime juice, and apple cider vinegar.

2. Muddle the lime wedges, mint leaves, and jalapeño slices in a shaker.

3. Add ice and pineapple puree to shaker. Shake vigorously.

4. Fill glasses with ice and divide the shaken mixture, including the muddled lime, mint leaves, and jalapeño slices, between the two glasses.

5. Top with seltzer and stir.

6. Garnish with mint sprigs, pineapple, or jalapeño slices (if you dare!).

FOR LESS HEAT, SWAP JALAPEÑO FOR CILANTRO OR CUCUMBER.

MOCKTAIL MULE

HIGHLIGHTS & BENEFITS
Hydrating ◆ May relieve nausea

Love the spicy taste of ginger in a drink but not the added sugar? Here, we show you an easy way to make your own "ginger juice" so you can control how much sugar you're putting in your drinks.

SERVES 2

INGREDIENTS

2 tsp fresh ginger, peeled and chopped

2 tbsp lime juice

½ cup coconut water

1–2 tsp light agave

¾ cup seltzer

Lime wedges for garnish

If you're experiencing a lot of nausea, leave the bit of ginger for extra relief.

TOOLS

Blender or food processor

Citrus Juicer

Strainer *(optional)*

PREPARATION

1. Blend coconut water, ginger, lime juice, and agave. Strain the mixture if your blender isn't able to get all the bits of ginger.

2. Divide mixture between glasses filled with ice.

Although this drink is pictured in a copper mug, know that acidic drinks can cause copper to leach from the cup into your drink. Instead, opt for a cermaic mug or one lined with stainless steel.

3. Top with seltzer and stir.

4. Garnish with lime wedges.

EXTRA GINGER? SEEP GINGER IN HOT WATER TO MAKE A GINGER TEA OR ADD IT TO AN ASIAN STIR-FRY DISH

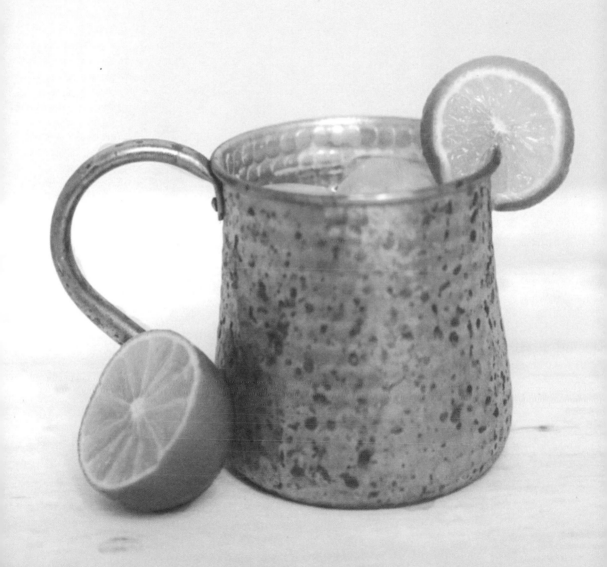

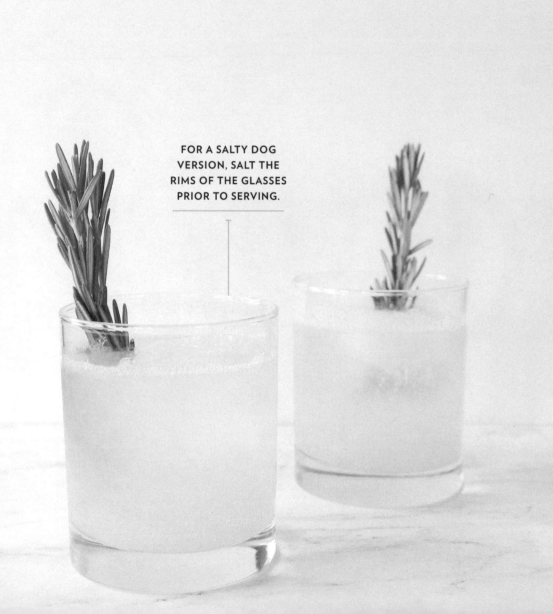

FOR A SALTY DOG
VERSION, SALT THE
RIMS OF THE GLASSES
PRIOR TO SERVING.

GRAPEFRUIT & ROSEMARY FIZZ

HIGHLIGHTS & BENEFITS

Hydrating • May relieve nausea • Naturally sweet • No added sugar

This citrus-heavy mocktail packs a vitamin C punch and is a fun fusion of a Greyhound and a classic Moscow Mule. The salt and rosemary add to the sensory experience, harmonizing the flavors and infusing a woodsy element.

SERVES 2

INGREDIENTS

½ cup grapefruit juice

2 tbsp lime juice

2 tsp fresh ginger, peeled and chopped

1 cup seltzer

1 dash salt per serving

2 rosemary sprigs for garnish

TOOLS

Blender or food processor

Citrus Juicer

PREPARATION

1. Blend the grapefruit juice, lime juice, salt, and ginger.

2. Divide the mixture between two glasses filled with ice.

3. Top with seltzer and stir.

4. Garnish with rosemary sprigs, swirling in the glass to infuse flavor.

USE EXTRA ROSEMARY ON ROASTED VEGETABLES LIKE BRUSSELS SPROUTS AND SWEET POTATO OR ATOP A PLAIN WHITE POTATO.

NATURALLY SHIRLEY

HIGHLIGHTS & BENEFITS

Contains antioxidants ◆ May relieve nausea ◆ Naturally sweet ◆ No sugar added

The classic non-alcoholic kid drink Shirley Temple is all grown up! We incorporated the flavors of the original concoction—grenadine and ginger ale—with the more familiar lemon & lime soda preparation of our generation. By swapping syrup for juice, you'll get an antioxidant boost without a sugar high.

SERVES 2

INGREDIENTS

⅔ cup 100% pomegranate juice (we like POM® brand)

¼ cup coconut water

2 tsp fresh ginger, peeled and chopped

1 lemon wedge

1 lime wedge

1 cup seltzer

Additional cherries for garnish

TOOLS

Blender or food processor

Muddler

Shaker

PREPARATION

1. Blend the ginger, pomegranate juice, and coconut water.

2. Muddle the lime and lemon wedges in the bottom of a shaker.

3. Add the blended mixture and ice to the shaker. Shake vigorously.

4. Divide the mixture between two ice-filled highball glasses.

5. Top with seltzer and stir.

6. Garnish with cherries.

EXTRA POMEGRANATE JUICE? TRY MAKING A POMEGRANATE SAUCE MARINADE FOR STEAK OR TOFU.

FESTIVE FIZZ

HIGHLIGHTS & BENEFITS
Contains antioxidants • May relieve nausea • Naturally sweet

Packed with seasonal flavors, like cranberry, citrus, and thyme, this mocktail is a perfect complement to your holiday dinner parties! Remember, mocktails are not just for pregnant women. Holidays are a time when people tend to go a little overboard with eating and drinking. Give your guests an alternative by offering a mocktail. They will thank you the next morning!

SERVES 2

INGREDIENTS

4 sprigs fresh thyme

2 tsp ginger, peeled and chopped

⅔ cup cranberry juice (see note below)

¼ cup and 2 tsbp orange juice

1 cup seltzer

Ice

Additional thyme and fresh cranberries for garnish

TOOLS

Muddler

Citrus Juicer

Shaker

PREPARATION

1. Muddle ginger and thyme in the bottom of a shaker.

2. Add the cranberry and orange juice; fill the shaker with ice. Shake vigorously.

3. Divide the shaken mixture between two ice-filled lowball glasses.

4. Top with seltzer and stir.

5. Garnish with thyme sprigs and fresh cranberries, if desired.

WE TESTED THIS RECIPE WITH THE MOST WIDELY AVAILABLE CRANBERRY JUICE, WHICH IS MIXED WITH WHITE GRAPE JUICE. YOU CAN FIND PURE 100% CRANBERRY JUICE AT HEALTH FOOD STORES AND EVEN SOME GROCERY STORES. IF YOU PREFER TO USE THIS, YOU MIGHT NEED TO DECREASE THE AMOUNT OF JUICE, CUT IT WITH SOME COCONUT WATER, AND/OR ADD A HINT OF LIGHT AGAVE TO YOUR DRINK, AS THE JUICE IS VERY TART ON ITS OWN.

BUBBLY DRINKS

GING-OSA

Ginger and apple cider vinegar add bite and tanginess to this mock mimosa. This drink goes well with brunch and self-care Sundays!

SERVES 2

INGREDIENTS

¾ cup of orange juice

For a fun variation, use blood orange juice or another citrus juice, like grapefruit.

2 tsp ginger, peeled and chopped

½ tsp apple cider vinegar

¾ cup seltzer *(more or less depending on how bubbly you like it)*

Orange slices and fresh thyme for garnish

TOOLS

Blender or food processor

Citrus Juicer

Shaker

PREPARATION

1. Blend ginger with apple cider vinegar and orange juice.

2. Add mixture to a shaker filled with ice. Shake vigorously.

3. Pour chilled mixture into champagne glasses.

4. Top with seltzer and stir.

5. Garnish with orange slices and fresh thyme.

ADD A SPLASH OF POMEGRANATE OR RED GRAPE JUICE (IN LIEU OF GRENADINE) TO MAKE A MOCK SUNRISE EFFECT.

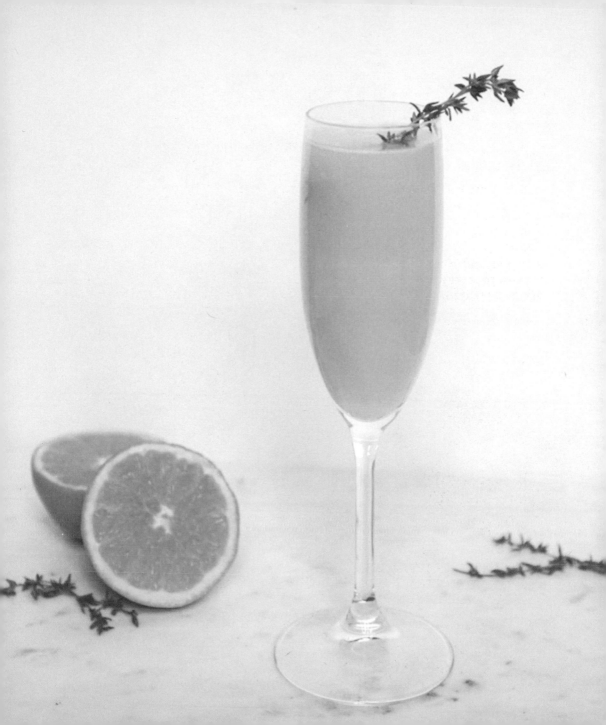

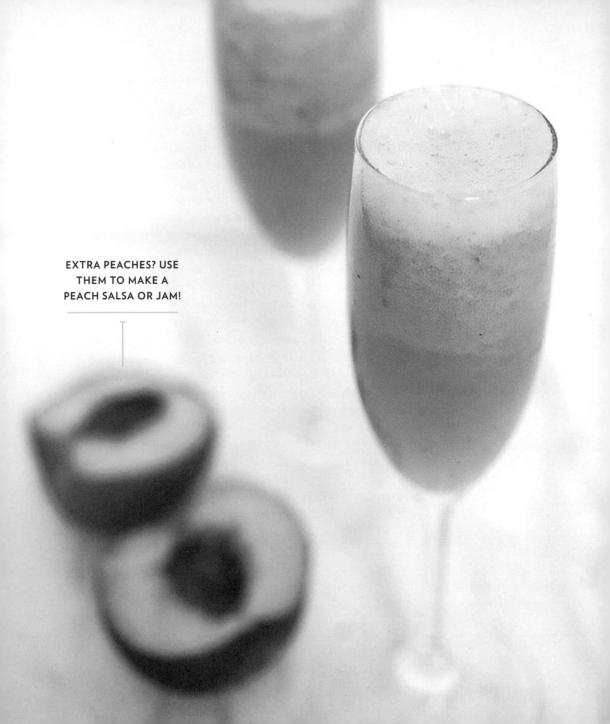

EXTRA PEACHES? USE
THEM TO MAKE A
PEACH SALSA OR JAM!

BELLY-NI

May relieve nausea ◆ Made with whole fruit ◆ Naturally sweet

We may have done away with the peach syrup in this Italian brunch staple,
but our version is just peachy!

SERVES 2

INGREDIENTS

1 medium peach, skin removed
*You may wish to blanch and cool the peach
to make it easier to remove the skin.*

¼ cup coconut water

1 pitted date

1 tbsp lemon juice

1 tsp apple cider vinegar

1 cup seltzer

TOOLS

Blender or food processor

Citrus Juicer

Shaker

Strainer *(optional)*

PREPARATION

1. Soak date for about 10 minutes.

2. Blend peach with lemon juice, apple cider vinegar, date, and coconut water until smooth.

3. Strain the mixture (if desired).

4. Pour mixture into shaker with ice. Shake vigorously.

5. Pour into champagne glasses. Top with chilled seltzer (approx. ½ cup in each cup), pouring slowly; stir gently.

YOU MAY NOTICE A SEPARATION IN THE DRINK AND A BUILD-UP OF FOAM WHEN YOU ADD THE SELTZER TO THE PUREE. FEAR NOT! THIS IS THE RESULT OF A REACTION BETWEEN THE FIBER IN THE PEACH AND THE CARBONATION. SIMPLY STIR THE DRINK TO HOMOGENIZE! OR, YOU CAN STRAIN THE PUREE BEFORE ADDING THE BUBBLES; THOUGH, THIS MAY DILUTE THE FLAVOR.

NO WAY ROSÉ

Rosé wine is all the rage nowadays. We created a non-alcoholic alternative that will satisfy your craving for a chilled and crisp glass of wine. The pomegranate and white grape juice provide the perfect rose color. In addition to vitamin C and vitamin E, pomegranate juice delivers folate, potassium, and vitamin K.

SERVES 2

INGREDIENTS

½ cup white grape juice

2 tbsp pomegranate juice

Cranberry juice or tart cherry juice would also be tasty!

½ cup coconut water

1 cup seltzer

1 tsp apple cider vinegar

1 tbsp lemon juice

TOOLS

Shaker

Citrus Juicer

PREPARATION

1. Add all ingredients (except seltzer) to a shaker filled with ice. Shake vigorously.

2. Pour into two wine glasses. Top with seltzer and stir.

USE LEFTOVER LEMON AND VINEGAR TO MAKE A FRUIT AND VEGETABLE WASH. MIX TOGETHER 1 TBSP LEMON JUICE, 2 TBSP VINEGAR, AND 1 CUP OF WATER.

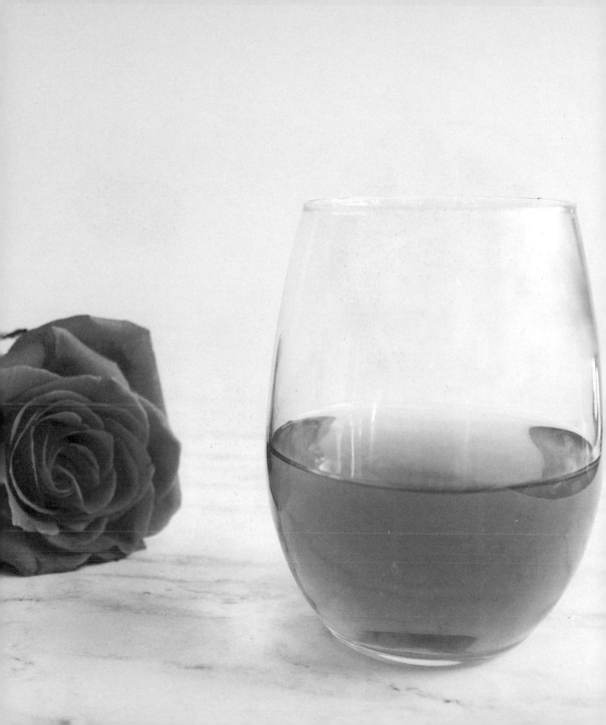

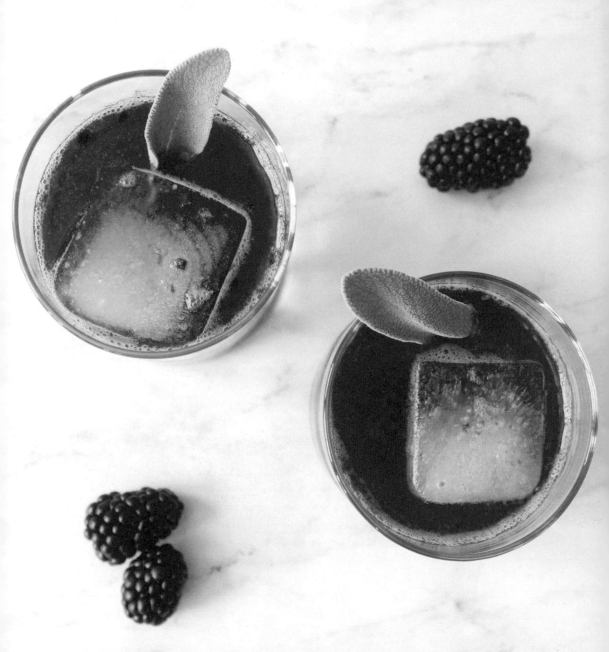

SMASHING SAGE SPRITZER

Muddled sage adds a unique, savory element that takes this drink to a new level. While you might associate this herb with Thanksgiving, this flavorful and vibrant mocktail would be perfect any time of the year.

SERVES 2

INGREDIENTS

1 cup fresh or frozen blackberries or cherries

1 tbsp lime juice

1 tsp honey

⅓ cup coconut water

1 cup seltzer

4 sage leaves

Additional blackberries and sage leaves for garnish

TOOLS

Muddler

Shaker

Citrus Juicer

PREPARATION

1. Muddle blackberries with sage leaves and honey in the bottom of a shaker.

2. Add lime juice and coconut water; fill shaker with ice. Shake vigorously. Strain, if desired.

3. Divide the shaken mixture between two ice-filled lowball glasses.

4. Top with seltzer and stir.

5. Garnish with fresh sage and blackberries.

Not a fan of sage? Substitute mint or other fresh herbs. You can easily adapt any of our recipes and play with different combinations of ingredients.

USE LEFTOVER SAGE TO ROAST WITH FRESH VEGETABLES. SAGE AND ROSEMARY PAIR WELL TOGETHER!

BUBBLY DRINKS

◆

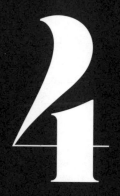

CHAPTER

4

FLAT
DRINKS

These flavorful drinks are perfect after the first trimester when nausea usually subsides. They also make an excellent option during preconception when you may be weaning yourself off of alcohol. For example, you can replace your nightly glass of wine or cocktails out on the town with our sophisticated sour recipe and fake out your friends and family. Many of these drinks contain fruit juices, which offer antioxidants and micronutrients, such as vitamin C. We even have a couple of vegetable-based recipes including beets and tomatoes!

BABY PALMER

HIGHLIGHTS & BENEFITS
Contains antioxidants • Hydrating

Just like the classic non-alcoholic Arnold Palmer you know and love, but with a twist—less sugar! This tangy beverage will keep you feeling refreshed on a hot summer day, perfect for outdoor grilling, picnics, and, of course, the golf course!

SERVES 2

INGREDIENTS

TEA
1 cup black tea (regular or decaf), brewed and cooled

LOW-SUGAR LEMONADE
¼ cup lemon juice

¾ cup coconut water

1 tbsp light agave nectar, or more if desired

Lemon wheels and mint for garnish

2 cups ice

TOOLS
Citrus Juicer

PREPARATION

PREPARE THE TEA
1. Boil water and steep with black tea of choice (we use Earl Grey) as directed on package. Allow to cool.

PREPARE THE LEMONADE
1. Mix the ingredients in a highball glass. Stir well.

PREPARE THE BABY PALMER:
1. Combine the lemonade and cooled tea.

2. Serve over ice immediately or allow to sit in the fridge for a few hours.

3. Garnish with lemon wheels and mint sprigs.

MAKE DOUBLE THE AMOUNT OF TEA, AND SAVE IT FOR THE NEXT DAY IF YOU WANT TO MAKE MINT-TEA JULEPS ON THE NEXT PAGE.

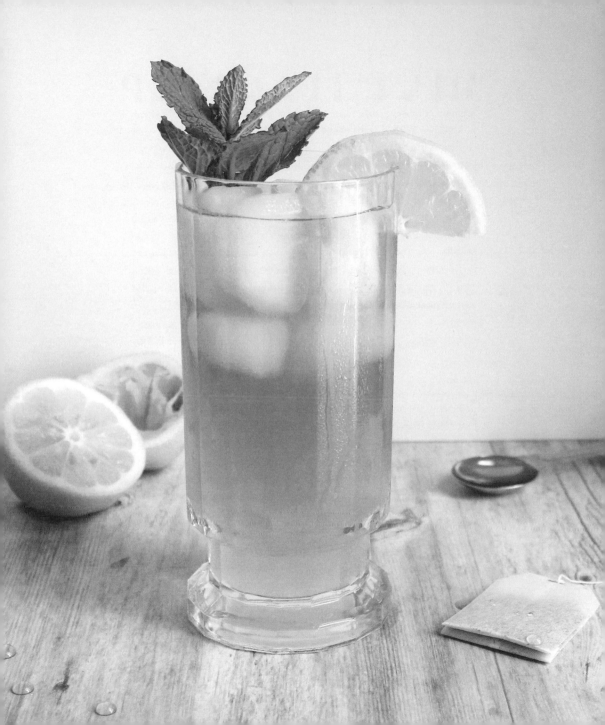

MINT-TEA JULEP

HIGHLIGHTS & BENEFITS
Contains antioxidants ◆ May relieve nausea

This mocktail is a very loose translation of the Kentucky Derby classic, the Mint Julep, which is traditionally made with whiskey, sugar, and mint. We substitute bourbon for black tea to mimic the look of this cocktail. No one has to know!

SERVES 2

INGREDIENTS

2 cups black tea (regular or decaf), brewed and cooled

15 mint leaves

4 slices each of lemon and lime

½ tsp apple cider vinegar

2 tsp light agave, if desired

Crushed ice

Additional mint for garnish

TOOLS

Muddler

PREPARATION

1. Boil water and steep with black tea of choice (we use Earl Grey) as directed on package. Allow to cool.

2. Muddle mint, agave, apple cider vinegar, lemon, and lime slices in the bottom of two mint julep cups.

Consider muddling ¼ cup fresh peach or apricot (per serving) with the mint!

3. Add crushed ice and pour cooled tea over the top. Stir well.

4. Garnish with mint sprig.

FOR A FRESH AND EARTHY TASTE, SWAP MINT FOR TARRAGON AND BLACK TEA FOR GREEN TEA. OR, SUBSTITUTE PLAIN BLACK TEA FOR 1 CUP OF OUR BABY PALMER RECIPE.

BEET-INI

HIGHLIGHTS & BENEFITS
Contains antioxidants • May relieve nausea • No added sugar

Squeezing in your veggies has never been simpler! This drink is vibrant in color and flavor, and for those of you who don't love beets, tastes sweet and nothing like them. Beets can change the color of your urine and stool, so don't be alarmed if you see some pink after you try this drink.

SERVES 2

INGREDIENTS

1 cooked baby beet, peeled and stemmed

1 medium apple, cored and chopped (we use Granny Smith)

1 tsp ginger, peeled and chopped

1 cup coconut water

¾ cup water

3 tbsp lemon juice

2 pitted dates

Lemon slices or lemon twist for garnish

TOOLS

Blender

Strainer or cheesecloth

Citrus Juicer

PREPARATION

1. Blend all ingredients and strain into an ice-filled shaker. Shake vigorously.

2. Serve in two martini glasses. Garnish with lemon slice or twist.

IN THIS RECIPE, YOU HAVE THE OPTION TO SHAKE WITH CHICKPEA LIQUID TO CREATE A FOAM EFFECT (SEE PAGE 82).

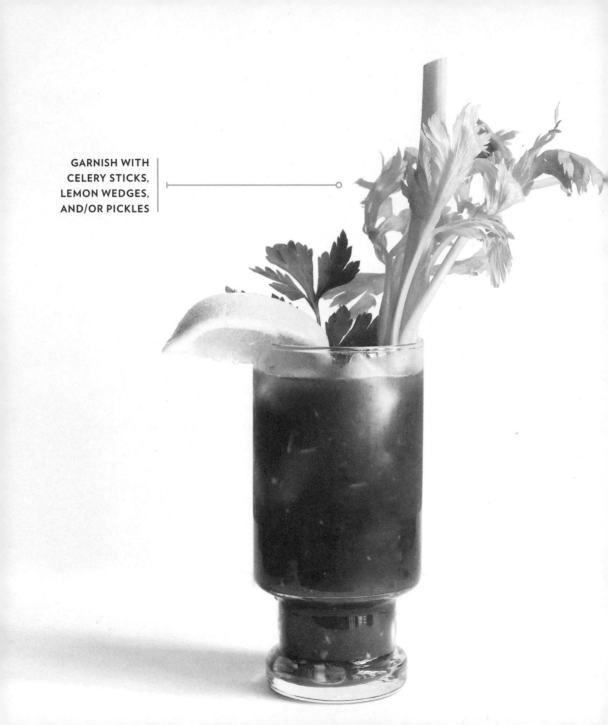

GARNISH WITH
CELERY STICKS,
LEMON WEDGES,
AND/OR PICKLES

VIRGIN MARY

HIGHLIGHTS & BENEFITS

Anti-aging ◆ Contains antioxidants ◆ Made with vegetables

This savory brunch classic has much more to offer than easing a hangover. Tomato is rich in vitamins C, A, B6, and potassium, as well as a powerful antioxidant called lycopene that has been linked to healthy aging (and prostate health). We like ours spicy, but this recipe is adaptable to your taste!

SERVES 2

INGREDIENTS

1 ½ cups prepared tomato juice or vegetable juice

We use low sodium tomato juice so that we can control the amount of salt.

⅓ cup dill pickle juice

1 tbsp lemon juice

1–2 tsp prepared horseradish, or as desired

¼–½ tsp hot sauce, or as desired

1 tsp Worcestershire sauce

Couple dashes salt (or seasoned salt)

¼ tsp freshly ground black pepper

Couple shakes cayenne pepper

Celery, lemon wedge, and pickle for garnish

Optional: jalapeño slices

TOOLS

Muddler

Shaker

Citrus Juicer

PREPARATION

1. Mix all of the ingredients (expect the jalapeño and garnishes) in the shaker and shake vigorously. Then, divide between two highball glasses. If desired, make ahead and chill overnight.

2. If using jalapeño, muddle in the bottom of two glasses before serving.

3. Garnish with celery, lemon wedge, and pickle.

SOUR GRAPES

This drink was inspired by the Pisco Sour, a cocktail that gets its name from the Peruvian spirit with which it is made. Many sour drinks contain raw egg white to add creaminess and a foam layer at the top of the drink. For a safer (and plant-based!) alternative, we subbed chickpea liquid, or aquafaba. Impress your guests and show off your skills by whipping up this sophisticated mocktail!

SERVES 2

INGREDIENTS

1 tbsp aquafaba
This is simply the liquid found in a can of chickpeas.

⅔ cup white grape juice

⅔ cup coconut water

¼ cup and 2 tbsp lime juice

Lime slices for garnish

TOOLS

Shaker

Citrus Juicer

PREPARATION

1. Dry shake (meaning: do not add ice) all ingredients in a shaker. Put some muscle into it!

2. Add ice. Shake vigorously a second time.

3. Serve in two lowball glasses.

4. Garnish with a slice of lime.

YES, WE KNOW ADDING CHICKPEA LIQUID TO A DRINK SOUNDS ODD, BUT WE PROMISE THE FUN FOAM EFFECT THAT IS CREATED IS ABSOLUTELY TASTELESS. THE ADDITION OF AQUAFABA AND THE TWO-STEP SHAKE TECHNIQUE CAN BE APPLIED TO OTHER DRINKS IN THIS BOOK—JUST AVOID SHAKING A CARBONATED DRINK! IN FACT, YOU CAN MAKE MANY THINGS WITH AQUAFABA. USING A MIXER, WHIP AQUAFABA WITH YOUR SWEETENER OF CHOICE TO MAKE A HEALTHIER MARSHMALLOW FLUFF!

PUCKER PUNCH

HIGHLIGHTS & BENEFITS

Contains antioxidants • Hydrating • May relieve nausea

This drink was inspired by a Boston Sour, which is simply a whiskey sour shaken with egg white, garnished with orange and a maraschino cherry. The ginger in our virgin version will not only replace the bite of the whiskey but also help alleviate nausea. Whip up this mocktail and your guests will never guess that you're sipping on something non-alcoholic!

SERVES 2

INGREDIENTS

1 tbsp aquafaba *(optional)*

¼ cup lemon juice

¼ cup pomegranate juice

1 cup coconut water

1 tsp fresh ginger, peeled and chopped (or ½ tsp apple cider vinegar)

Orange slices and cherries for garnish

TOOLS

Shaker

Citrus Juicer

Muddler

PREPARATION

1. Muddle ginger in the bottom of a shaker.

2. Add the remaining ingredients. Dry shake vigorously for 1 minute.

3. Add ice. Shake vigorously for another 30 seconds.

4. Serve over ice in lowball glasses.

5. Garnish with a slice of orange and sweet or maraschino cherry.

IF YOU HAVE EXTRA POMEGRANATE JUICE, IT CAN BE ADDED TO SOME GREEK YOGURT FOR A TASTY POMEGRANATE YOGURT SAUCE TO ADD TO SALADS OR AS A DIP!

SOUR MOCK-A-RITA

Love a good, strong margarita but not the sugar & alcohol headache it gives you the next morning? We have the solution! This hydrating version uses coconut water instead of tequila and keeps the added sugar to a minimum. A perfect complement to tacos or chips & guacamole!

SERVES 2

INGREDIENTS

SALTED RIM
Lime wedges

Sea salt

DRINK
½ cup and 1 tbsp lime juice

3 tbsp orange juice

1 ½ tsp light agave nectar

1 ¼ cups and 1 tbsp coconut water

2 cups ice

Couple dashes of salt

TOOLS
Shaker

Citrus Juicer

PREPARATION
1. Salt the rims of the serving glasses.

DRINK
1. In a shaker, combine juice, agave, salt, and coconut water with ice. Shake vigorously.

2. Pour into lowball glasses over ice.

THROW IN FRESH OR FROZEN FRUIT BEFORE BLENDING FOR NATURAL SWEETNESS—YOU MAY NOT EVEN NEED THE AGAVE!

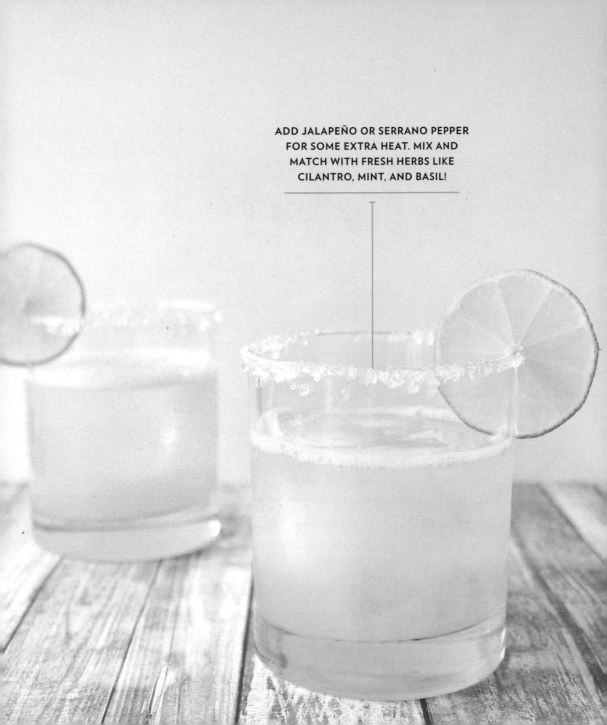

ADD JALAPEÑO OR SERRANO PEPPER FOR SOME EXTRA HEAT. MIX AND MATCH WITH FRESH HERBS LIKE CILANTRO, MINT, AND BASIL!

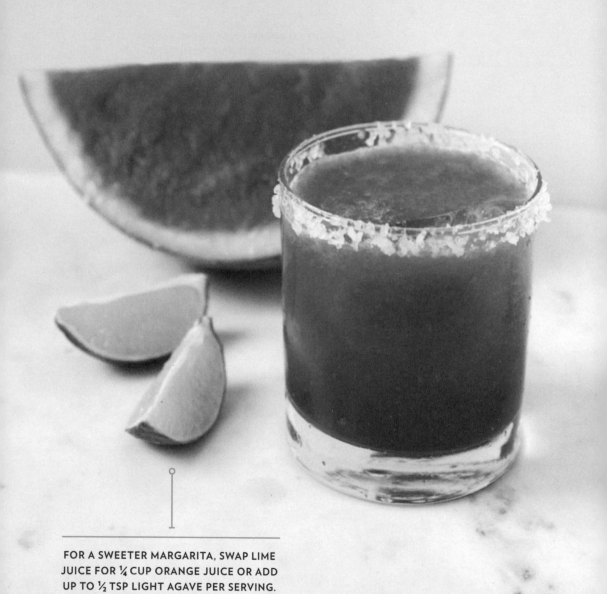

FOR A SWEETER MARGARITA, SWAP LIME JUICE FOR ¼ CUP ORANGE JUICE OR ADD UP TO ½ TSP LIGHT AGAVE PER SERVING.

WATERMELON MOCK-A-RITA

HIGHLIGHTS & BENEFITS

Hydrating • Made with whole fruit • Naturally sweet

This mock-a-rita, made with coconut water and watermelon, is ultra-hydrating and super refreshing. Watermelon is also high in an amino acid called citrulline, which can actually help relax blood vessels and lower blood pressure.

SERVES 2

INGREDIENTS

SALTED RIM
Lime wedges
Sea salt

DRINK
1 ½ cups fresh watermelon, seeds removed
¼ cup lime juice
½ cup coconut water
Dash of salt
2 cups ice
Watermelon slices for garnish

TOOLS

Shaker
Citrus Juicer
Blender or food processor

PREPARATION

1. Salt the rims of the serving glasses.

2. Blend watermelon until it forms a juice.

3. In a shaker, combine watermelon juice, lime juice, salt, and coconut water. Add ice and shake vigorously.

4. Serve in lowball glasses over ice.

5. Garnish with watermelon slices.

THIS DRINK CAN BE PREPARED AS A "SHAKEN" COCKTAIL AND SERVED OVER ICE, AS ABOVE, OR BLENDED WITH ICE FOR A FROZEN TREAT! IF YOU WANT AN EARTHIER VERSION WITH ADDED NUTRITIONAL VALUE, TRY ADDING 1 TSP CILANTRO PER SERVING. CILANTRO CONTAINS VITAMINS A AND K, POTASSIUM, AND FOLATE.

SPICY CUCUMBER MOCK-A-RITA

HIGHLIGHTS & BENEFITS
Boosts metabolism ◆ Hydrating

The cool cucumber provides sweet relief from the heat of the jalapeño in this mock margarita. Feel free to adjust either flavor to hit the right balance for your palate!

SERVES 2

INGREDIENTS

SALTED RIM
Lime wedges

Sea salt

DRINK
8 slices of cucumber

¼ cup + 2 tbsp lime juice

2 tbsp orange juice

Jalapeño slices (as many as you dare, but 1–2 will do the trick. Remove seeds and membrane to tone down the heat)

2 tsp light agave nectar

¾ cup coconut water

2 cups ice

1–2 dashes salt

Cucumber and jalapeño slices for garnish

TOOLS
Shaker

Muddler

Citrus Juicer

PREPARATION

1. Salt the rims of the serving glasses.

2. Muddle cucumber and jalapeño with agave in the bottom of a shaker.

3. Add lime juice, orange juice, salt, and coconut water.

4. Add ice and shake vigorously.

5. Pour into salt rimmed lowball glasses over ice, including muddled cucumber and jalapeño (if desired).

6. Garnish with cucumber and jalapeño slices.

EXTRA CUCUMBER? TRY MAKING A GREEK-INSPIRED CUCUMBER, TOMATO, AND FETA SALAD (BE SURE THE CHEESE HAS BEEN PASTEURIZED).

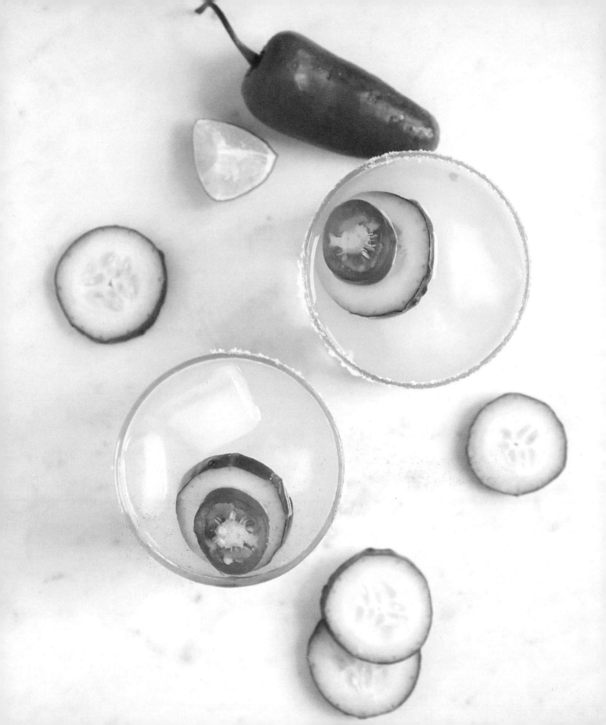

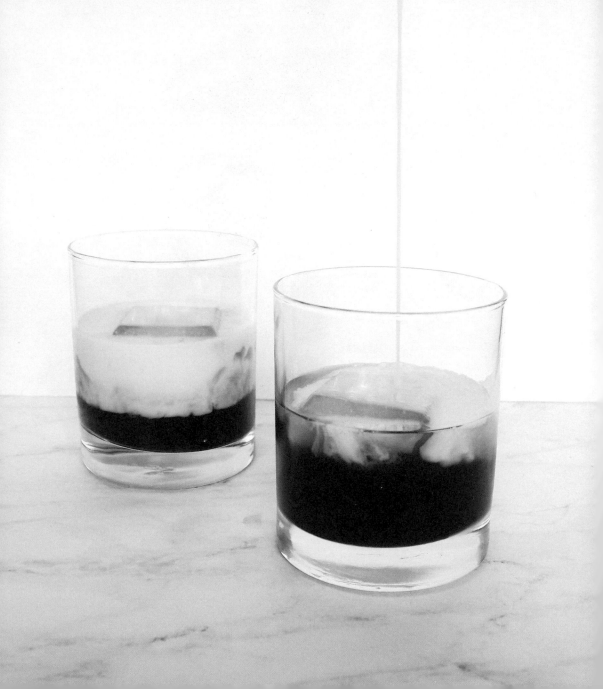

WHITE-ISH RUSSIAN

HIGHLIGHTS & BENEFITS
Provides an energy boost ◆ Satisfies sweet cravings

Coconut cream gives our non-alcoholic White Russian the rich, creamy texture of the original. Perfect for when you've got a hankering for some coffee but you're trying to cut back—there's only two ounces per serving!

SERVES 2

INGREDIENTS

¼ cup coconut milk (canned)

¼ cup non-dairy milk

½ cup coffee (regular or decaf), brewed and cooled

Make your life easier and purchase a cold brew!

1 tsp non-alcoholic vanilla extract
Conventional pure vanilla extract contains alcohol, so we recommend using a non-alcoholic version.

1–2 tsp sweetener (maple syrup or light agave work well)

We recommend using 2 tsp of sweetener if you are using strong coffee.

TOOLS

Shaker

Food processor *(optional)*

PREPARATION

1. Shake canned coconut milk before opening. You can also blend the coconut milk in a food processor to make sure it's well-mixed.

2. In a shaker with ice, combine coffee, vanilla, and sweetener.

3. Divide the mixture between two ice-filled lowball glasses.

4. Combine coconut cream and nondairy mix in the shaker; pour the mixture in slowly for a layered effect.

LEFTOVER COCONUT MILK CAN BE USED IN MANY OF THE OTHER DRINKS IN THIS BOOK, OR YOU CAN USE IT IN MANY CURRY RECIPES OR TO MAKE COCONUT WHIPPED CREAM!

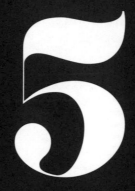

CHAPTER

5

FROZEN
DRINKS

The drinks in the following chapter are made with whole fruit (and even vegetables!) whenever possible, so you get fiber along with nutrients. In addition, these drinks are more substantial and are an appropriate and nutritious way to increase your calorie intake as you progress through your pregnancy. In contrast to the alcoholic versions of these drinks, the use of whole fruit and hydrating coconut water will help prevent a blood sugar spike.

STRAWBERRY BASIL VIRGIN DAQUIRI

HIGHLIGHTS & BENEFITS

Contains antioxidants • Contains fiber for digestive health
Made with whole fruit and vegetables • Naturally sweet

We added basil to this classic frozen drink for flavor and function, as it is thought to have antimicrobial and anti-inflammatory effects, among other health benefits. We also added frozen cauliflower rice to give this drink extra creaminess and additional nutrients—we promise you won't taste it!

SERVES 2

INGREDIENTS

2 cups frozen strawberries

Pick the reddest strawberries for even more sweetness. Don't use sweetened berries (added sugar!).

12 small fresh basil leaves

1 tbsp lemon juice

3 pitted dates

1 ½ cups coconut water

½ cup frozen cauliflower rice

1 cup ice

Additional basil leaves and sliced strawberries for garnish

TOOLS

Blender

Citrus Juicer

PREPARATION

1. Soak dates in water for 10 minutes.

2. Place strawberries, lemon juice, coconut water, dates, cauliflower rice, basil, and ice into blender.

3. Blend on high for a longer period of time to break up the dates for evenly distributed sweetness.

4. Garnish with fresh basil and sliced strawberries.

FROZEN TEQUILA-LESS SUNRISE

HIGHLIGHTS & BENEFITS
Contains fiber for digestive health • Made with whole fruit • Naturally sweet

Although the flavors may be different from a classic Tequila Sunrise, made with orange juice and grenadine, you'll still get the beautiful sunrise colors in this tasty mocktail. Each layer has a unique taste, but the real magic happens when you mix the two together. A perfect poolside beverage!

SERVES 2

INGREDIENTS

FOR LAYER 1
1 cup frozen mango
¾ cup coconut water
1 tbsp lime juice
¾–1 cup ice

FOR LAYER 2
1 cup frozen strawberries
¾ cup coconut water
1 tbsp lime juice
2 pitted dates
¾–1 cup ice
Lime slices for garnish

TOOLS

Blender

Citrus Juicer

PREPARATION

1. Soak dates in water for 10 minutes.

2. Add Layer 1 ingredients to blender.

3. Blend until smooth, and then place in the freezer to keep cold.

4. Meanwhile, add Layer 2 ingredients to blender.

5. Blend until smooth.

6. Serve by pouring alternating flavors in the glasses to create a layered effect.

7. Garnish with lime slices.

CHIPOTLE MANGO VIRGIN DAQUIRI

HIGHLIGHTS & BENEFITS:

Contains fiber for digestive health • Made with whole fruit • Naturally sweet

We combined chipotle, lime, and mango to bring you a unique set of flavors. The mango adds sweetness, the lime brings the tanginess, and the chipotle delivers the kick! Feeling a little backed up? Then this tropical mocktail is definitely for you. Mango contains fiber and has a high water content, both of which will help move things along.

SERVES 2

INGREDIENTS

2 cups frozen mango

Don't use sweetened mango (added sugar!).

2 tbsp lime juice

1 ½ cups coconut water

1 pitted date

¼ tsp chipotle powder

½ cup ice

Additional mango and chipotle powder for garnish

TOOLS

Blender

Citrus Juicer

PREPARATION

1. Soak the date in water for 10 minutes.

2. Add all ingredients to a blender.

3. Blend on high for a longer period of time to break up the date for evenly distributed sweetness.

4. Garnish with extra mango pieces and a dash of chipotle powder.

DID YOU KNOW THAT WHEN YOU STRIP DOWN THE MARGARITA AND DAQUIRI TO THEIR MOST BASIC PREPARATIONS, THEY DIFFER ONLY IN THE TYPE OF LIQUOR USED (RUM VERSUS TEQUILA)?

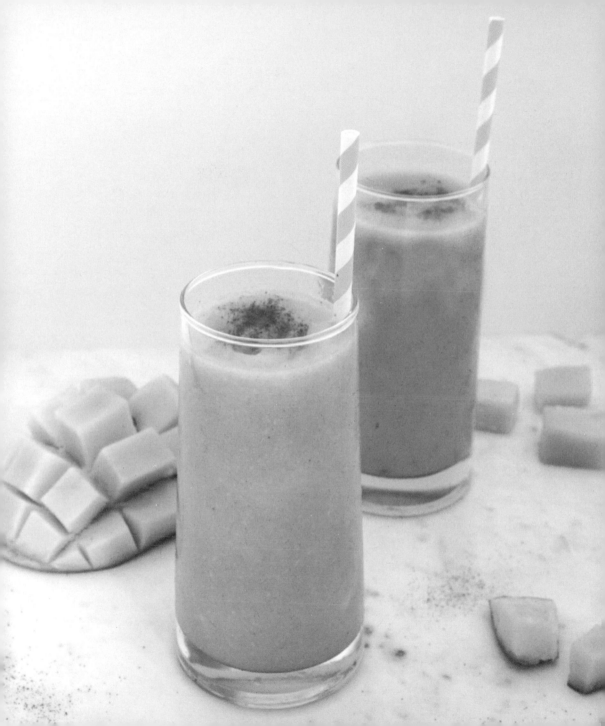

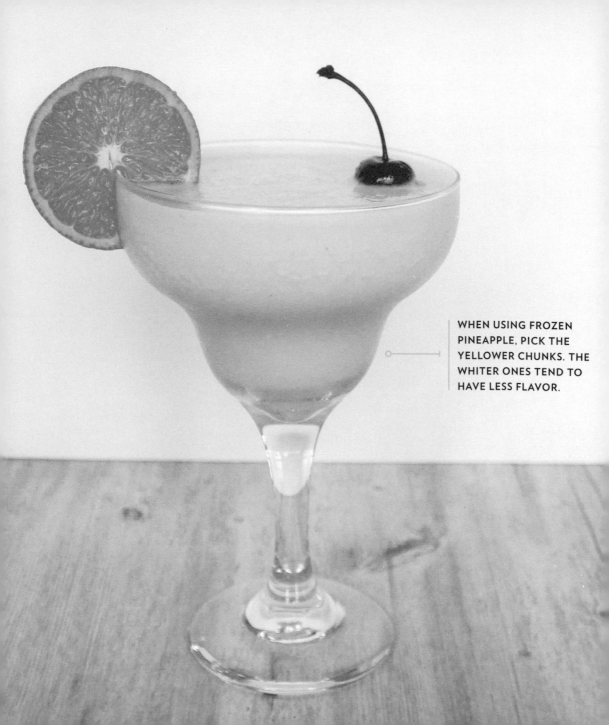

WHEN USING FROZEN PINEAPPLE, PICK THE YELLOWER CHUNKS. THE WHITER ONES TEND TO HAVE LESS FLAVOR.

PIÑA COL-NADA

HIGHLIGHTS & BENEFITS

Contains fiber for digestive health ◆ Made with whole fruit and vegetables

Transport yourself to paradise in seconds with our take on a Piña Colada. This sweet, frozen treat captures the essence of the original, but we use frozen cauliflower to enhance creaminess, making this drink a great way to sneak in some veggies!

SERVES 2

INGREDIENTS

2 cups frozen pineapple

1 cup unsweetened coconut milk (carton) (use more if needed to facilitate blending)

¼ cup coconut milk (canned)

½ cup frozen cauliflower or cauliflower rice

We highly recommend using frozen cauliflower!

Squeeze of fresh lime juice

Pineapple or orange slices and sweet cherries for garnish

TOOLS

Blender

PREPARATION

1. Add all ingredients to blender.

2. Blend on high until smooth and frothy.

3. Garnish with pineapple, orange slices, or maraschino cherries.

BE SURE TO STICK WITH FROZEN FRUIT FOR THIS RECIPE. IF YOU HAVE FRESH FRUIT ON HAND, FREEZE IT AHEAD OF TIME OR BE SURE TO ADD A LOT OF ICE (1- 2 CUPS) TO THE RECIPE TO MAKE IT THE RIGHT CONSISTENCY. KEEPING IN MIND THAT THIS WILL INCREASE THE QUANTITY MADE (BY UP TO TWO SERVINGS).

MOCHA-NUT

HIGHLIGHTS & BENEFITS

Naturally sweet ◆ Provides an energy boost ◆ Satisfies sweet cravings

Inspired by a frozen mudslide cocktail, which is made with coffee-flavored liqueur, Irish cream, and vodka, this drink is a much more nutritious way to satisfy your craving for a blended coffee beverage or chocolate treat. The cacao used in this recipe is what chocolate is made from. It contains fiber, iron, magnesium, and antioxidants.

SERVES 2

INGREDIENTS

1 cup non-dairy milk

½ cup coconut milk (canned)

2 ½ tbsp brewed espresso or coffee (can be decaf)

1 tsp non-alcoholic vanilla extract

1–2 tbsp unsweetened cocoa or cacao powder

3 pitted dates

2 cups ice

Cacao nibs, chocolate chips, or coconut whipped cream for garnish

Optional: try adding 1 tbsp of flax or chia seeds for extra omega 3s.

TOOLS

Blender

PREPARATION

1. Soak dates in water for 10 minutes.

2. Add all ingredients to a blender.

3. Blend on high for a longer period of time to break up dates for evenly distributed sweetness.

4. Garnish with cacao nibs, chocolate chips, or a dollop of coconut whipped cream.

TO MAKE COCONUT WHIPPED CREAM

1. Refrigerate full fat canned coconut milk overnight.

2. Scoop out thickened cream from can and place in a mixing bowl. Discard any excess liquid. Add a touch of maple syrup if desired.

3. Using a hand mixer, whip coconut cream until desired fluffiness is reached (around 3-5 minutes).

DID YOU KNOW THAT LIGHT ROASTS ACTUALLY HAVE MORE CAFFEINE THAN DARK ROASTED COFFEES?

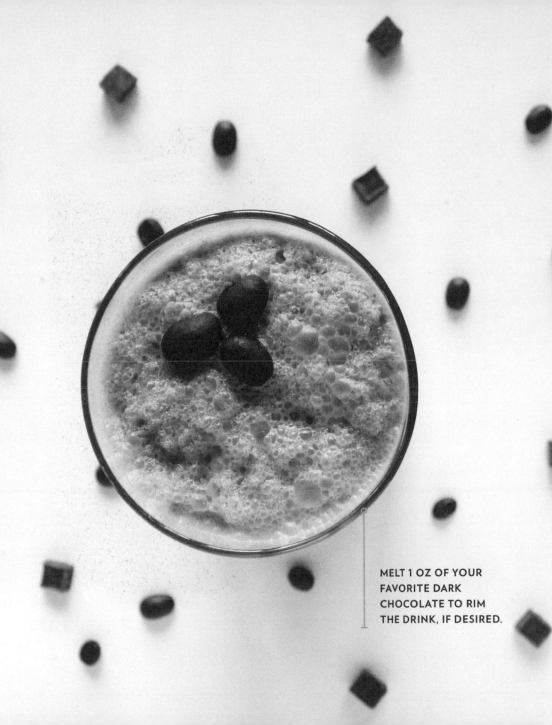

MELT 1 OZ OF YOUR
FAVORITE DARK
CHOCOLATE TO RIM
THE DRINK, IF DESIRED.

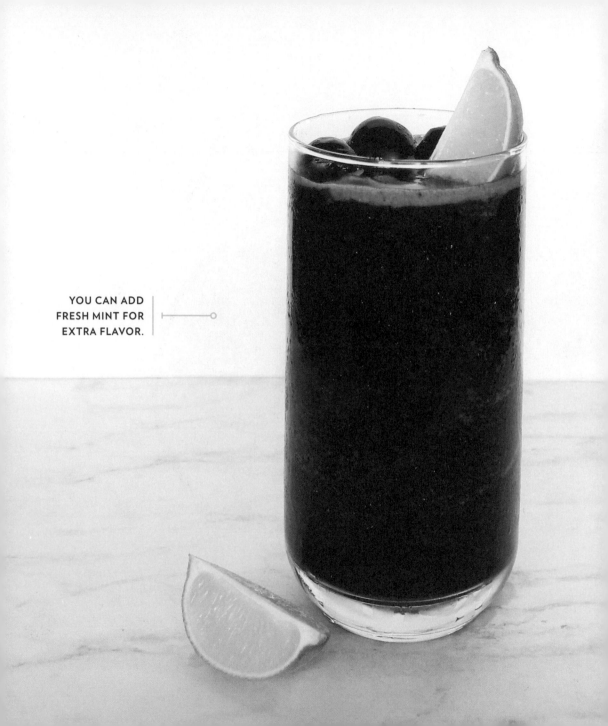

YOU CAN ADD
FRESH MINT FOR
EXTRA FLAVOR.

FROZEN CHERRY LIMEADE

HIGHLIGHTS & BENEFITS

Contains fiber for digestive health • Made with whole fruit • Naturally sweet

A frozen twist on the fast-food classic, our cherry limeade uses fruit and fresh-squeezed juices to make a sweet and tart treat, avoiding concentrated juices and syrups, sugar, and soda.

SERVES 2

INGREDIENTS

2 cups frozen or fresh sweet cherries (add ½ cup of ice if using fresh cherries)

1 cup coconut water

3 tbsp lime juice

2 tbsp orange juice

Lime wedges and additional cherries for garnish

TOOLS

Blender

Citrus Juicer

PREPARATION

1. Add all ingredients to a blender.

2. Blend on high until the ingredients are well mixed.

3. Garnish with extra cherries and lime wedges.

IF YOU HAVE EXTRA CHERRIES, YOU CAN MAKE YOUR OWN BERRY OR CHERRY COMPOTE TO SERVE WITH PANCAKES OR WAFFLES. HEAT 2 CUPS OF FRUIT IN A SAUCEPAN UNTIL THE JUICES START TO WEEP FROM THE FRUIT. THEN ADD 1-2 TBSP OF CHIA SEEDS, ALONG WITH A SQUEEZE OF FRESH LEMON JUICE AND, IF DESIRED, 1 TSP OF HONEY OR MAPLE SYRUP.

FROZEN COS-NO-POLITAN

You'll love this frozen, tart, and alcohol-free take on the Cosmopolitan: the classic city girl's cocktail! Cranberries are chock-full of antioxidants, including vitamin C, which helps keep your skin looking youthful and radiant and prevents stretch marks.

SERVES 2

INGREDIENTS
2 cups frozen cranberries

1 tbsp lime juice

¼ cup orange juice

1 ½ cups coconut water

3–4 pitted dates

1 cup of ice

TOOLS
Citrus Juicer

Blender

PREPARATION
1. Soak the dates in water for 10 minutes.

2. Add all ingredients to a blender.

3. Blend on high for a longer period of time to break up the dates for evenly distributed sweetness.

4. Serve in martini glasses.

EXTRA CRANBERRIES? WHIP UP A SIMPLE CRANBERRY SAUCE FOR YOUR NEXT SANDWICH! TIP: USE FRESHLY SQUEEZED ORANGE JUICE INSTEAD OF SUGAR.

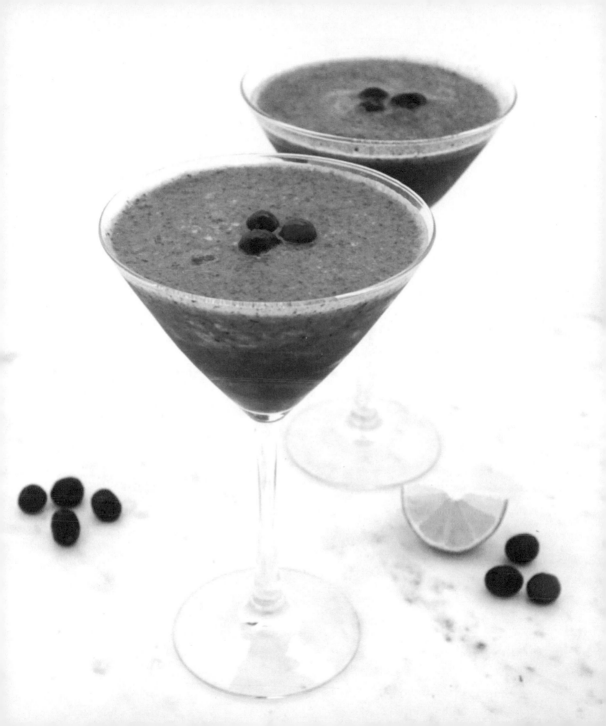

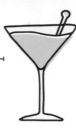

MOCK-TINI

DRINKS

◆

These drinks are a little more decadent but still packed with nutrition. Like the frozen drinks, mock-tinis can increase your energy intake in a healthy and nutritious way—and will hopefully satisfy your sweet cravings! Since many of these drinks contain nut milks and nuts, we provide guidance for allergy-friendly, plant-based alternatives. The use of dried fruit, namely in the form of dates, provides fiber and nutrients like iron, important during the second half of pregnancy. Other sweeteners used are chosen for their appropriateness in the drink but also nutritional value. For example, molasses is high in B6 and iron!

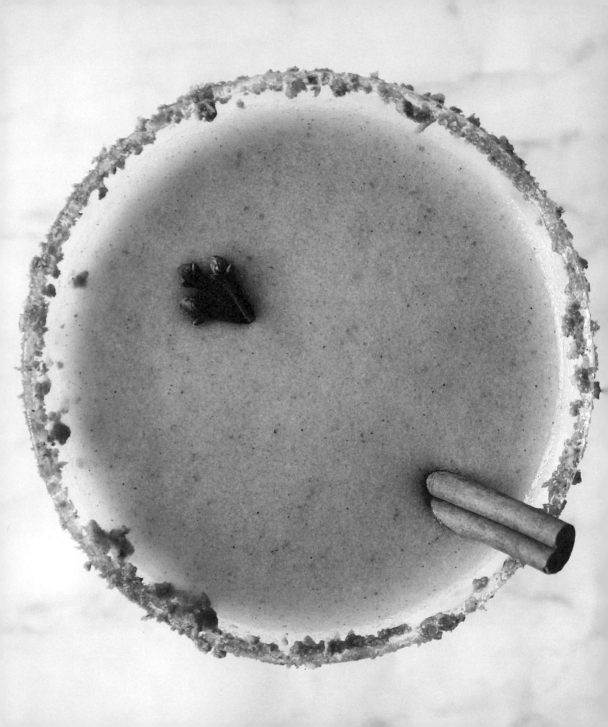

APPLE PIE MOCK-TINI

HIGHLIGHTS AND BENEFITS

Contains fiber for digestive health ◆ Naturally sweet

Applesauce in a drink? Don't knock it until you try it! Inspired by the classic, all-American dessert, we captured the warm, fall spices in apple pie and made a nutritious mocktail that delivers soluble fiber and vitamin C. To get the real feel of fresh baked apple pie, you can even try this concoction warm!

SERVES 2

INGREDIENTS

RIM

1 tbsp chopped nuts or ground graham crackers

1 tsp maple syrup or honey

DRINKS

1 cup unsweetened applesauce (or about 2 standard single-serve containers)

You can also swap for 100% apple juice.

2 pitted dates

1 cup coconut water

¼ tsp ground cinnamon

2 shakes ground nutmeg

1 shake ground cloves

1 tbsp lemon or lime juice

½ tsp non-alcoholic vanilla extract

Apple slices or cinnamon stick for garnish

TOOLS

Blender or food processor

Citrus Juicer

Shaker

PREPARATION

1. Soak dates in water for 10 minutes.

2. Meanwhile, rim glasses with maple syrup or honey and then dip into ground nuts or graham crackers.

3. Add the dates and applesauce to a blender.

4. Blend on high for a longer period of time to break up the dates for evenly distributed sweetness.

5. Add the mixture and remaining ingredients to a shaker with ice. Shake vigorously.

Skip this step if you want to try the warm version.

6. Pour into martini glasses and garnish with a slice of fresh apple or a cinnamon stick.

THROW A DOLLOP OF FROZEN YOGURT OR NON-DAIRY VANILLA ICE CREAM ON TOP!

MOCK-TINI DRINKS

◆

PUMPKIN PIE MOCK-TINI

HIGHLIGHTS & BENEFITS

Contains fiber for digestive health • Made with vegetables • Nutrient-dense

Just like a slice of your favorite Thanksgiving pie, this martini goes down smooth and spicy. It's decadent like pumpkin pie filling and can even be eaten with a spoon! Canned pumpkin delivers a healthy dose of fiber, magnesium and vitamins A, C, and K.

SERVES 2

INGREDIENTS

PUMPKIN PIE RIM

1 tbsp chopped walnuts

Use graham crackers for a nut-free version!

1 tsp maple syrup

DRINK

1 ½ cups non-dairy milk

⅔ cup canned pure pumpkin puree (not pumpkin pie filling)

3–4 pitted dates

1 ½ tsp pumpkin pie spice

½ tsp non-alcoholic vanilla extract

Pinch of salt

Coconut whipped cream (refer to page 100 for recipe) and ground cinnamon for garnish

TOOLS

Blender or food processor

PREPARATION

1. Soak dates in water for 10 minutes.

2. Meanwhile, rim glasses with maple syrup and then dip into chopped walnuts.

3. Add all ingredients to a blender.

4. Blend on high for a longer period of time to break up the dates for evenly distributed sweetness.

5. Pour into prepared martini glasses.

6. Garnish with a dollop of coconut whipped cream and a sprinkle of cinnamon.

EXTRA CANNED PUMPKIN? TRY MAKING PUMPKIN CHOCOLATE CHIP ENERGY BALLS. OR MAKE YOUR OWN PUMPKIN SOUP!

MOCK-TINI DRINKS

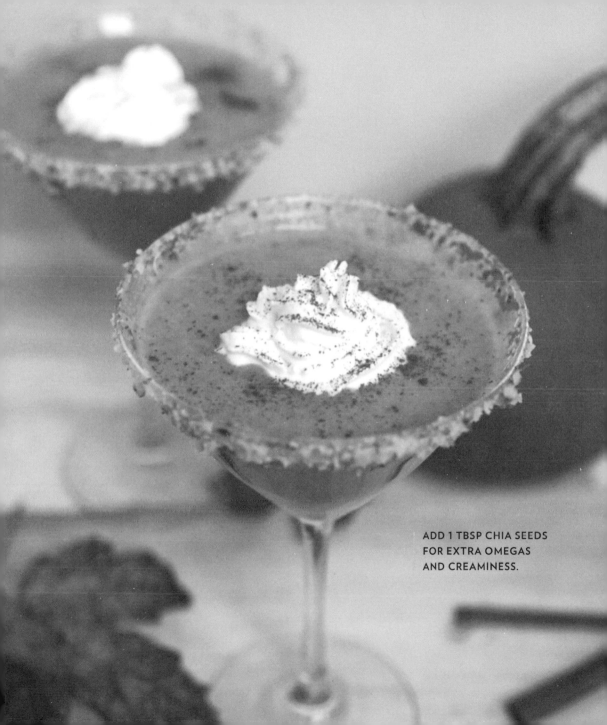

ADD 1 TBSP CHIA SEEDS
FOR EXTRA OMEGAS
AND CREAMINESS.

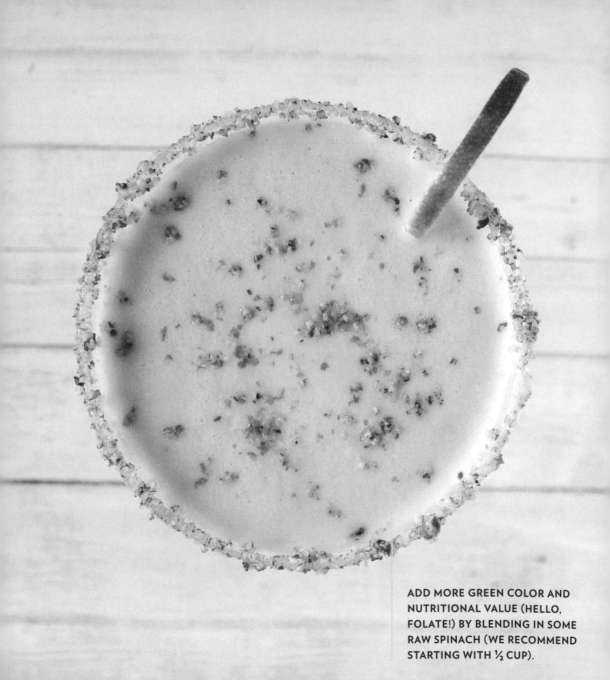

ADD MORE GREEN COLOR AND NUTRITIONAL VALUE (HELLO, FOLATE!) BY BLENDING IN SOME RAW SPINACH (WE RECOMMEND STARTING WITH ½ CUP).

KEY LIME PIE MOCK-TINI

HIGHLIGHTS & BENEFITS
Contains fiber for digestive health ◆ Made with whole fruit ◆ Naturally sweet

Just like the classic southern dessert, this Key Lime Pie Mock-tini is the perfect balance of sweet and tart. We transformed this decadent dessert into a nutrient-dense mocktail, and our version gets its sweetness naturally from pineapple and dates rather than sweetened condensed milk.

SERVES 2

INGREDIENTS

KEY LIME PIE RIM

1 tbsp walnuts, almonds, or pecans, finely ground

For a nut-free version, use graham cracker.

1 tsp maple syrup

DRINK

2 cups fresh or frozen pineapple

1 cup non-dairy milk

¼ cup key lime juice

You can use regular lime juice if you can't find key limes!

1 pitted date

1 tsp non-alcoholic vanilla extract

Key lime slices and ground nuts for garnish

Pinch of salt

TOOLS

Blender or food processor

Citrus Juicer

PREPARATION

1. Soak dates in water for 10 minutes.

2. Meanwhile, wet the rims of martini glasses with maple syrup and then dip into crushed nuts.

3. Add all ingredients to a blender.

4. Blend on high for a longer period of time to break up the dates for evenly distributed sweetness.

5. Pour into martini glasses and serve with a lime slice and a sprinkling of ground nuts.

BANANA CREAM PIE
MOCK-TINI

HIGHLIGHTS & BENEFITS

Contains fiber for digestive health ◆ Contains healthy fats ◆ Provides a boost of potassium

Ripe bananas make this recipe extra sweet, smooth, and fluffy. Their high potassium content can help replenish lost electrolytes from morning sickness.

SERVES 2

INGREDIENTS

BANANA CREAM PIE RIM

2 tbsp walnuts or almonds, finely grounded

For a nut-free version, use graham cracker.

1 tbsp maple syrup

DRINK

1 cup non-dairy milk

2 ripe bananas (the riper the better!)

⅓ cup cashews, soaked for 6 hours or overnight

For nut free version, sub equivalent amount of coconut milk (canned).

1 tsp non-alcoholic vanilla extract

1 pitted date

Pinch of salt

Banana slices and coconut whipped cream (refer to page 100 for recipe)

Optional: add 1 tbsp of chia seeds for extra omegas and creaminess.

TOOLS

Blender or food processor

PREPARATION

1. Soak date in water for 10 minutes.

2. Meanwhile, wet the rims of two martini glasses with maple syrup and then dip into nuts.

3. Add all ingredients to a blender.

4. Blend on high for a longer period of time to break up the dates for evenly distributed sweetness.

5. Pour into martini glasses and garnish with sliced banana and a dollop of coconut whipped cream.

MILK OR COOKIES MOCK-TINI

HIGHLIGHTS & BENEFITS

Satisfies sweet cravings • Provides a boost of iron

Molasses is packed with nutrients, including magnesium, iron, and B6, and is low in sugar relative to other sweeteners. We got two different vibes from this drink: is it gingerbread, or does it taste like cinnamon-flavored cereal milk?

SERVES 2

INGREDIENTS

COOKIE RIM

1 tbsp finely ground nuts, gingerbread cookies, or graham crackers

1 tsp maple syrup

DRINK

1 ½ cups non-dairy milk

½ tsp non-alcoholic vanilla extract

¼ cup coconut milk (canned)

1 ½ tbsp blackstrap molasses

1 tsp fresh ginger, peeled and chopped

½ tsp cinnamon

Pinch of nutmeg

Pinch of ground cloves

Pinch of salt

Crumbled gingerbread cookies or nuts for garnish

TOOLS

Blender or food processor

Strainer (*optional*)

PREPARATION

1. Rim two glasses with maple syrup and then dip into ground cookies or nuts.

2. Add all ingredients to the blender.

3. Blend well until the ingredients look smooth and creamy.

4. If desired, strain any remaining bits of ginger.

5. Pour into martini glasses and garnish with crumbled gingerbread cookies or nuts.

LEFTOVER MOLASSES CAN BE USED IN BARBECUE OR GINGERBREAD RECIPES.

MOCK-TINI DRINKS

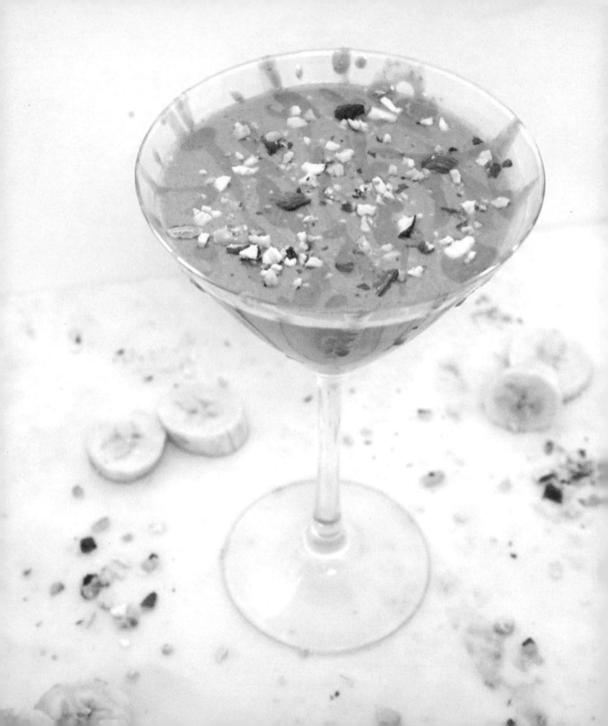

FUNKY MONKEY MOCK-TINI

HIGHLIGHTS & BENEFITS

Contains fiber for digestive health ◆ Contains healthy fats
Satisfies sweet cravings

Peanut butter cups meet banana and chocolate chunk ice cream! This mocktail has a healthy dose of peanut butter which is high in a healthy fat known as monounsaturated fat. This drink will satisfy a sweet tooth and also keep you feeling full.

SERVES 2

INGREDIENTS

1 ½ cups non-dairy milk

¼ cup natural peanut butter (or your favorite nut, seed, or soy butter)

1 ripe banana

½ tsp non-alcoholic vanilla extract

2 tsp unsweetened cocoa or cacao powder

Sprinkle of sea salt

Crushed nuts for garnish

Optional: Add chia seeds for omega 3's, fiber, and added creaminess! The chia seeds absorb liquid and can be added to many of our mock-tini and frozen drinks for a thicker (and more nutritious) beverage!

TOOLS

Blender or food processor

PREPARATION

1. Add all ingredients to a blender.

2. Blend well until the contents look smooth and frothy.

3. Pour into martini glasses and garnish with crushed nuts.

YOU CAN FREEZE THE BANANA AHEAD OF TIME FOR A THICKER FROZEN TREAT. IF YOU DON'T LIKE BANANAS OR ARE ALLERGIC TO THEM, FEEL FREE TO SUBSTITUTE TWO DATES.

CHOCOLATE CREAM MOCK-TINI

HIGHLIGHTS & BENEFITS
Contains fiber for digestive health • Contains healthy fats
Provides a boost of iron • Satisfies sweet cravings

If you have a craving for chocolate, then this is the recipe for you! Dark chocolate can be an excellent source of iron, providing up to 30% of the recommended daily value. It is also full of flavonoids—antioxidant compounds that help fight inflammation. This chocolate cream martini gets its decadent, mousse-like consistency from a secret ingredient—avocado! We promise you won't taste it; instead you get a rich, creamy dessert beverage.

SERVES 2

INGREDIENTS

RIM
1 oz dark chocolate, melted

DRINK
2 cups non-dairy milk

1 ½-oz dark chocolate, melted

¼ cup avocado

For an avocado-free version, use ½ cup canned coconut milk.

1 tsp non-alcoholic vanilla extract

3 pitted dates

2 tbsp unsweetened cocoa powder or cacao powder

Pinch of salt

Optional: add 1 tbsp flax or chia seeds for extra omega 3's.

TOOLS

Blender or food processor

PREPARATION

1. Soak dates in water for 10 minutes.

2. Meanwhile, rim glasses by dipping them in melted chocolate.

3. Allow chocolate to harden by placing glasses in the refrigerator for 10 minutes.

4. Add all ingredients to a blender.

5. Blend on high for a longer period of time to break up the dates for evenly distributed sweetness.

6. Pour into chilled martini glasses.

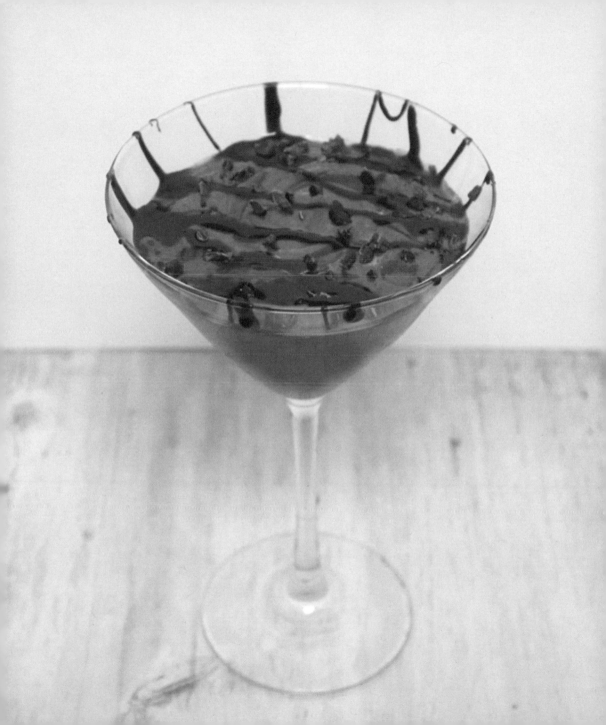

CHAPTER

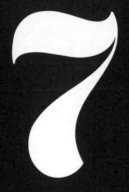

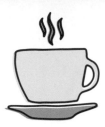

WARM

DRINKS

You'll notice that many of our warm drinks are inspired by beverages that are already non-alcoholic (with the exception of our "Not Toddy"). Instead, we focused on creating healthier, nutrient-dense versions of classic cool weather drinks, like apple cider and hot chocolate, as well as less traditional drinks, like our Soothing Spiced Latte. Flavorful and functional, these cozy concoctions will warm you from the inside out and help you survive the winter blues!

INSTANT CIDER

HIGHLIGHTS & BENEFITS
Contains fiber for digestive health • No added sugar

What could be more perfect than a glass of hot apple cider on a crisp fall day? We came up with a shortcut method that will shave hours off the prep time. Interestingly, some pre-made ciders are technically juices, meaning that they have been filtered. A true cider is unfiltered and may also be unpasteurized; though, most if not all commercial ciders are now pasteurized. If you purchase cider, always double check the label to see if it is pasteurized and doesn't contain added sugars. As we address in Appendix 2 (page 148), pasteurization is important, because it kills potentially harmful bacteria.

SERVES 2

INGREDIENTS

1 ½ cups 100% apple juice

1 cup coconut water

¼ tsp cinnamon

2 cinnamon sticks

1 tsp ginger, peeled and chopped

2 tbsp orange juice

1 tsp apple cider vinegar

Additional cinnamon sticks, whole cloves, or apple slices for garnish

TOOLS

Blender

Citrus Juicer

PREPARATION

1. Add all ingredients (except cinnamon sticks) to a blender.

2. Blend until smooth.

3. Strain out any residual ginger bits, if desired.

4. Heat the blended mixture along with the cinnamon sticks on the stovetop.

You can eliminate this step and serve this drink cold!

5. Serve in mugs.

6. Garnish with cinnamon sticks or whole cloves.

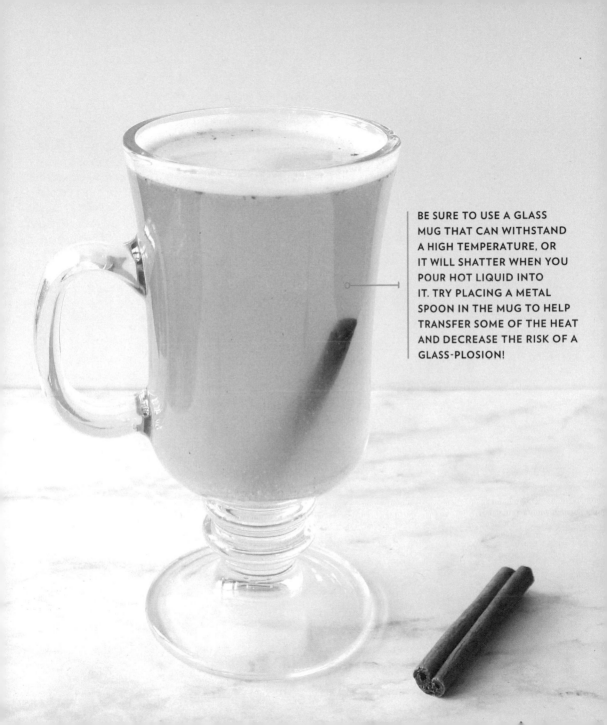

BE SURE TO USE A GLASS
MUG THAT CAN WITHSTAND
A HIGH TEMPERATURE, OR
IT WILL SHATTER WHEN YOU
POUR HOT LIQUID INTO
IT. TRY PLACING A METAL
SPOON IN THE MUG TO HELP
TRANSFER SOME OF THE HEAT
AND DECREASE THE RISK OF A
GLASS-PLOSION!

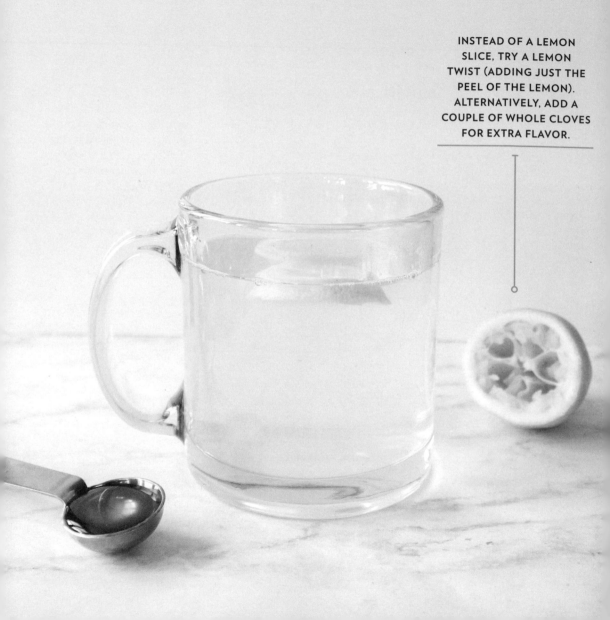

INSTEAD OF A LEMON
SLICE, TRY A LEMON
TWIST (ADDING JUST THE
PEEL OF THE LEMON).
ALTERNATIVELY, ADD A
COUPLE OF WHOLE CLOVES
FOR EXTRA FLAVOR.

NOT-TODDY

A perfect restorative beverage for cold & flu season

A traditional hot toddy is a soul-soothing cocktail made with just four ingredients: whiskey, lemon, honey, and hot water. In our mocktail, we use apple cider vinegar to mimic the bite of whiskey in the original and to add some additional sweetness. Feel free to tweak the proportions to your taste preferences!

SERVES 2

INGREDIENTS

3 cups boiling water

1½ tbsp lemon juice

1½ tbsp apple cider vinegar

2 tsp honey

Cinnamon sticks and lemon slices for garnish

TOOLS

Citrus Juicer

PREPARATION

1. Divide lemon juice, apple cider vinegar, and honey between two mugs.

2. Pour hot water into the mugs.

3. Serve with a cinnamon stick and a slice of lemon.

BOIL HALF OF AN APPLE WITH THE WATER TO MAKE AN APPLE NOT-TODDY

COLD-KICKER ELIXIR

HIGHLIGHTS & BENEFITS
A perfect restorative beverage for cold & flu season

This is our tried and true recipe for beating a cold before it takes hold. Start sipping on this at the first sign of malaise and repeat as needed!

SERVES 2

INGREDIENTS

2 cups boiling water

Few slices of fresh ginger (peeled, if desired)

2 bags black or green tea (regular or decaf)

You can even omit the tea!

2 slices of lemon

1–2 tsp honey, as desired

Pinch of cayenne pepper

Additional lemon slices for garnish

TOOLS

None!

PREPARATION

1. Prepare the tea: boil water with ginger slices, and then brew with tea bags and lemon slices.

Tip for reducing the caffeine content of tea: steep for a few minutes and then re-use the tea bag to brew the tea you'll use in your drink.

2. Add honey and cayenne.

3. Serve with a slice of fresh lemon.

SPICED LATTE

HIGHLIGHTS & BENEFITS
Anti-inflammatory ◆ Contains antioxidants

This coconut milk latte is warming, spicy, and nutrient-rich. Turmeric contains curcumin, a phytonutrient with many reported health benefits, namely reducing inflammation. The black pepper and the fat in the canned coconut milk may help facilitate absorption of turmeric. Both ingredients also contribute to the mouthfeel of the drink, with coconut milk for creaminess and black pepper for heat.

As with other herbs & spices, turmeric is likely safe to consume during pregnancy in amounts commonly used in cooking but not in a supplemental or "medicinal" dose. As always, check with your doctor before adding anything new to your diet or supplement regimen.

SERVES 2

INGREDIENTS

½ cup coconut milk (canned)

1 ¾ cups non-dairy milk

½ tsp non-alcoholic vanilla extract

1 tbsp honey, light agave or maple syrup

¼ tsp ground turmeric

You can omit the turmeric, if desired.

½ tsp pumpkin spice

⅛ tsp ground ginger

¼ tsp ground cinnamon, plus more for garnish

2 dashes black pepper

Extra ground cinnamon or cinnamon sticks for garnish

TOOLS

None!

PREPARATION

1. Place the coconut milk, non-dairy milk, sweetener, and non-alcoholic vanilla extract in a saucepan and slowly bring to a simmer.

2. Add the spices to the saucepan. Whisk mixture until ingredients are well combined.

Use a frother to add a foam effect!

3. Simmer for 3–5 minutes.

4. Pour into mugs and garnish with extra cinnamon or a cinnamon stick.

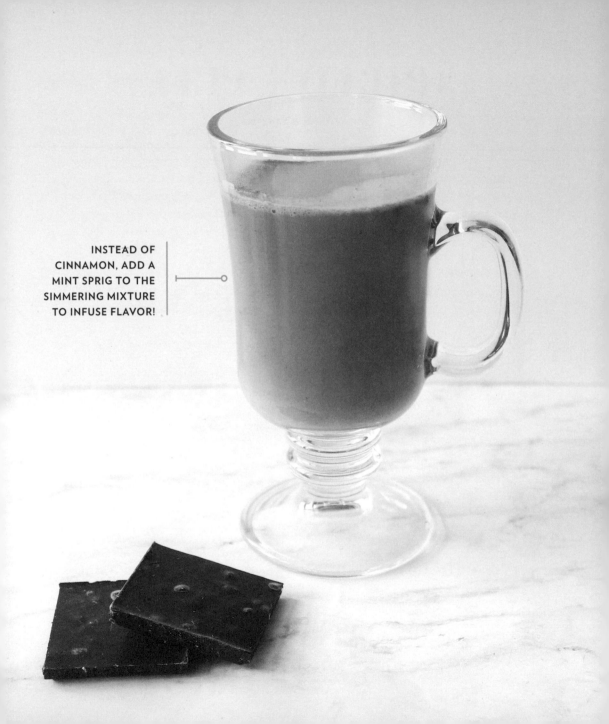

INSTEAD OF CINNAMON, ADD A MINT SPRIG TO THE SIMMERING MIXTURE TO INFUSE FLAVOR!

PLANT-BASED HOT CHOCOLATE

HIGHLIGHTS & BENEFITS
Provides a boost of iron ◆ Satisfies sweet cravings

Nothing beats a mug of velvety hot chocolate on a chilly, snowy winter night! Cozy up by the fire with our antioxidant-rich, low sugar, plant-based version. You can easily adjust the intensity of the chocolate to your taste in two ways: with the percent cacao of your dark chocolate and the amount of sweetener that you add. Not that we need an excuse to eat more chocolate, but it does have nutritional value! Dark chocolate, depending on the intensity, contains iron, fiber, and antioxidants. The higher the percent cacao, the greater the benefits. Chocolate does contain saturated fat, though, and thus should be enjoyed in moderation. We've found that with bitter, dark chocolate, it is easier to keep the portions in check.

SERVES 2

INGREDIENTS

1½ oz dark chocolate

½ cup coconut milk (canned)

1 ¾ cups non-dairy milk

1–2 tbsp maple syrup or light agave nectar

1 tbsp unsweetened cocoa powder or cacao powder

½ vanilla bean, split lengthwise or 1 tsp non-alcoholic vanilla extract

¼ teaspoon sea salt

¼ tsp cinnamon

Coconut whipped cream for garnish (refer to page 100 for recipe)

Optional: add a pinch of cayenne for a Mexican hot chocolate

TOOLS

None!

PREPARATION

1. Place the dark chocolate, coconut milk, non-dairy milk, desired syrup, vanilla bean, and sea salt in a saucepan and slowly bring to a simmer as you stir. Don't allow the liquid to come to a boil, as this will impact the flavor of the chocolate and cocoa powder.

2. Add the cocoa powder and cinnamon to the saucepan. Whisk until the mixture is combined.

3. Simmer for 3–5 minutes.

4. Taste hot chocolate and add more syrup or nectar if you desire a sweeter drink.

5. Pour into mugs and top with coconut whipped cream.

WARM DRINKS

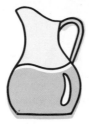

BATCH
DRINKS

I n this chapter, we provide you with batch recipes perfect for dinner parties, holidays, and special occasions like baby showers, Mother's Day, and gender reveal parties, to name a few! The recipes in this chapter make 6-8 servings of drinks that are traditionally served in larger quantities, like sangria, punch, and lemonade. Of course, you can double or triple these recipes for larger parties, or you can scale up any of the drinks from previous chapters. Share your nutrition knowledge and spread the health benefits around!

RED SANS-GRIA

Our mock red sangria recipe is simple, naturally sweet, and easily adapted to your tastes and to the occasion. For example, you can add a few cinnamon sticks and cloves for some fall flair, or throw in some fresh herbs, like rosemary, thyme, or mint.

SERVES 6

INGREDIENTS

2 ½ cups pomegranate juice (no sugar added) or grape juice (or a combination of the two!) *A small amount of tart cherry juice would give this a bit of an edge!*

2 ½ cups coconut water

1 cup orange juice

¼ cup lime juice

1 lemon thinly sliced, with peel

1 lime thinly sliced, with peel

1 medium orange thinly sliced, with peel

1 small apple cored, sliced into eighths, with peel

TOOLS

Muddler

Citrus Juicer

PREPARATION

1. Add sliced fruit to a large pitcher. Muddle.

2. Add the pomegranate, coconut water, and citrus juices. Stir well.

3. Place in refrigerator and let chill for at least 3–4 hours.

4. Serve over ice in highball glasses, including the fruit.

FUN FACT: POMEGRANATE JUICE HAS THE HIGHEST ANTIOXIDANT PROFILE OF ANY JUICE, AND MANY EVEN TRUMP WINE!

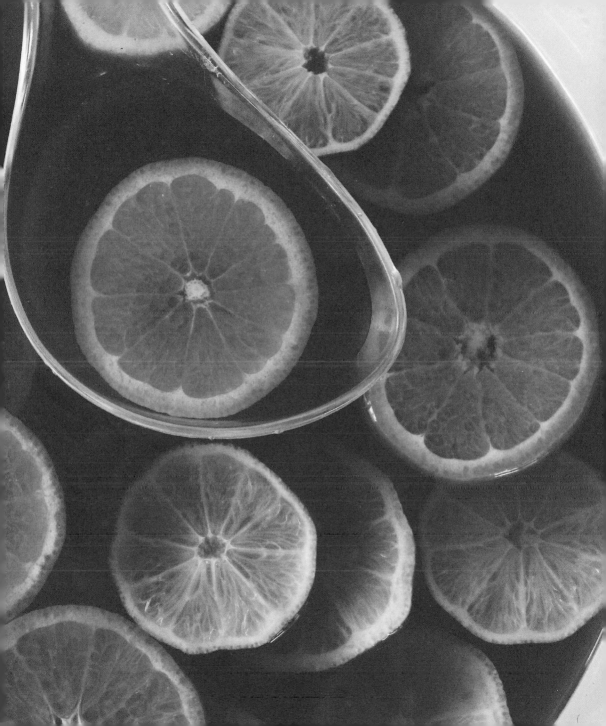

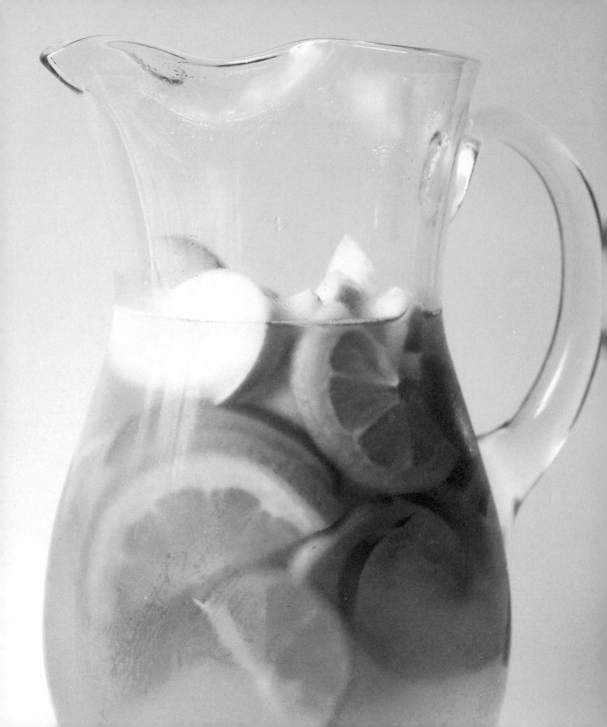

WHITE SANS-GRIA

Our non-alcoholic white sangria is light and perfect for summer gatherings. Feel free to get creative with your additions. Blue and red berries would be adorable for a gender reveal party!

SERVES 6

INGREDIENTS
2 ½ cups white grape juice

2 ½ cups coconut water

¼ cup lime juice

1 lemon thinly sliced, with peel

1 lime thinly sliced, with peel

1 medium orange thinly sliced, with peel

½ grapefruit, sliced

½ peach, sliced

1 can club soda (or 12 ounces)

Mint and club soda to garnish

Optional. additional club soda for serving

TOOLS
Muddler

Citrus Juicer

PREPARATION
1. Add sliced fruit to a large pitcher. Muddle.

2. Add the white grape juice, coconut water, and lime juice. Stir well.

3. Place in refrigerator and let chill for 3-4 hours.

4. When ready to serve, top with club soda. Stir well.

5. Serve over ice in highball glasses, including the fruit.

6. Garnish with fresh mint and top with additional club soda, if desired.

MULLED WINE-NOT

HIGHLIGHTS & BENEFITS
Contains antioxidants

This cozy mocktail is the hot counterpart to our red sans-gria. With wintry spices like cinnamon and clove, it will warm you from the inside out.

SERVES 6

INGREDIENTS

3 cups pomegranate juice (no sugar added) or grape juice

3 cups coconut water

½ cup orange juice

Zest of ½ orange

Zest of ½ lemon

12 whole cloves

4 cinnamon sticks

¼ tsp ground nutmeg

¼ tsp ground cardamom

Lemon and orange slices and cinnamon sticks for garnish

Optional: up to 1 tbsp honey; up to 3 star anise pods (licorice flavor)

TOOLS

Citrus Juicer

PREPARATION

1. Simmer pomegranate and citrus juices, coconut water, honey (if using), spices, cloves, and zest for 15 minutes over low heat. Avoid boiling the mixture.

2. Serve with fresh lemon slices, orange slices, and cinnamon sticks.

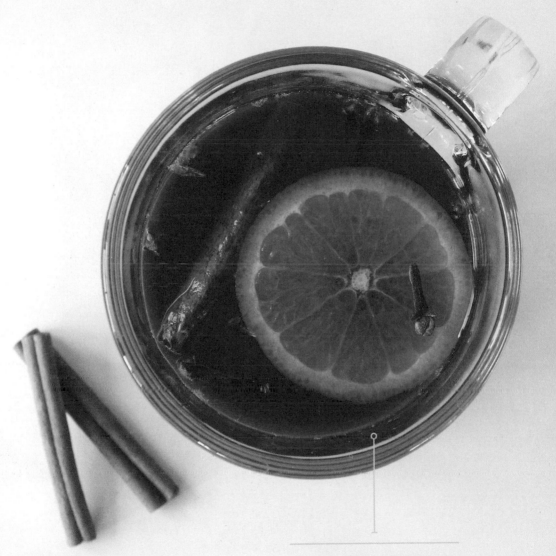

USE 100% APPLE JUICE TO MAKE
YOUR OWN NO SUGAR-ADDED
MULLED CIDER!

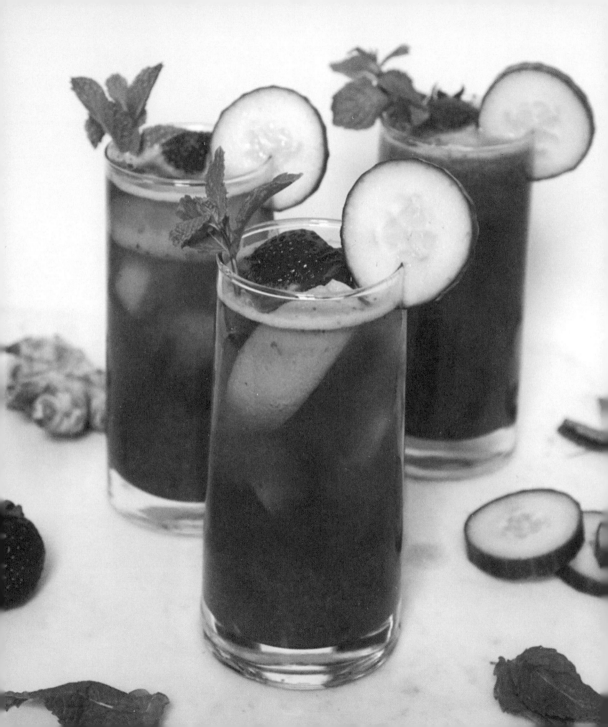

BRITISH BREW

HIGHLIGHTS & BENEFITS
Hydrating

The Pimm's Cup is a classic British cocktail that is herbaceous and fruity. Our alcohol-free version captures the complexity of the original—no two sips taste the same! The cucumber is cool and refreshing, perfect for outdoor activities or watching Wimbledon.

SERVES 4-6

INGREDIENTS

6 slices of cucumber, plus more for garnish

12 large strawberries, plus more for garnish

3 cups black tea, brewed with 4–5 mint leaves and cooled

Decaf or regular depending on your desired caffeine intake.

3 cups coconut water, blended with a small piece of fresh ginger and 1 tbsp balsamic vinegar

Juice of 1 lemon and 1 lime (2 tbsp of each)

1 ½ cups seltzer

Cucumber, lemon, strawberries, rosemary, thyme, or mint for garnish

Optional: 1½ tsp light agave nectar

TOOLS

Blender or food processor

Muddler

Citrus Juicer

PREPARATION

1. Muddle cucumber and strawberries in the bottom of a pitcher.

2. Add brewed tea, blended coconut water, citrus juice, and agave. Stir well.

3. Place in refrigerator and let chill for 3–4 hours.

4. When ready to serve, top with club soda. Stir well.

5. Serve over ice in highball glasses.

6. Garnish with cucumber slices, lemon slices, fresh strawberries, and sprigs of fresh rosemary, thyme, or mint, as desired.

HAVE EXTRA HERBS? CHOP AND MAKE HERB ICE CUBES TO USE LATER! FOR A VARIATION TO THIS DRINK, PREPARE WITH 1 CUP OF OUR BABY PALMER RECIPE (PAGE 76) INSTEAD OF TEA.

SOFT LEMONADE

HIGHLIGHTS & BENEFITS
Contains antioxidants ◆ Hydrating

We softened the calorie and sugar blow that comes with traditional and hard lemonades with our lower sugar version. Filled with seltzer and hydrating coconut water, this thirst-quenching mix is perfect for outdoor parties and BBQs on a hot summer day.

SERVES 6

INGREDIENTS
¾ cup lemon juice

3 cups coconut water

3 tbsp light agave nectar

3 cups seltzer

Lemon slices for garnish

TOOLS
Citrus Juicer

PREPARATION

1. Mix the lemon juice, coconut water, and agave nectar in a pitcher. Stir well.

2. Top with seltzer; stir.

3. Serve over ice in highball glasses.

4. Garnish with lemon slices.

SLUSH PUNCH

HIGHLIGHTS & BENEFITS
Anti-inflammatory • Hydrating

Punches are dangerously good but can be shockingly high in alcohol and sugar. Our version incorporates whole fruit in the form of pineapple, hydrating coconut water, and tart cherry juice, which is antioxidant-rich and has been shown to help with muscle recovery after intense physical activity. Talk about a punch of nutrients!

SERVES 6

INGREDIENTS

3 cups tart cherry juice

2 cups frozen pineapple

2 cups coconut water

3 tbsp lime juice

1 lemon, thinly sliced with peel

1 lime, thinly sliced with peel

1 medium orange thinly sliced, with peel

2 cups ice

Pineapple or orange slices and cherries for garnish

TOOLS

Blender

Citrus Juicer

PREPARATION

1. Add sliced fruit to a large pitcher. Muddle.

2. Blend pineapple, cherry juice, coconut water, lime juice, and ice.

3. Add blended juice to pitcher.

4. If desired, place in freezer and let chill further for 1–2 hours.

5. When ready to serve, stir punch and pour into highball glasses.

6. Garnish with cucumber slices, lemon slices, fresh strawberries, and sprigs of fresh rosemary, thyme, or mint, as desired.

EGGLESS-NOG

Traditional eggnog is brimming with heavy cream and sugar. Our goal was to create a healthier version without sacrificing taste and mouthfeel. The coconut milk provides the consistency while the dates deliver the sweetness. This combination will not only satisfy your craving for eggnog around the holidays but also keep you feeling full.

SERVES 6

INGREDIENTS

6 cups non-dairy milk

We recommend almond, oat, or soy milk.

1 ½ cups coconut milk (canned)

1 ½ tsp non-alcoholic vanilla extract

¼ tsp nutmeg

⅛ tsp cinnamon

6 pitted dates

Ground nutmeg or cinnamon for garnish

TOOLS

Blender

This may need to be done in batches depending on how much liquid your blender holds.

PREPARATION

1. Soak dates for 10 minutes.

2. Blend the dates well, then add the rest of the ingredients and blend again.

3. Serve with a sprinkle of nutmeg or cinnamon.

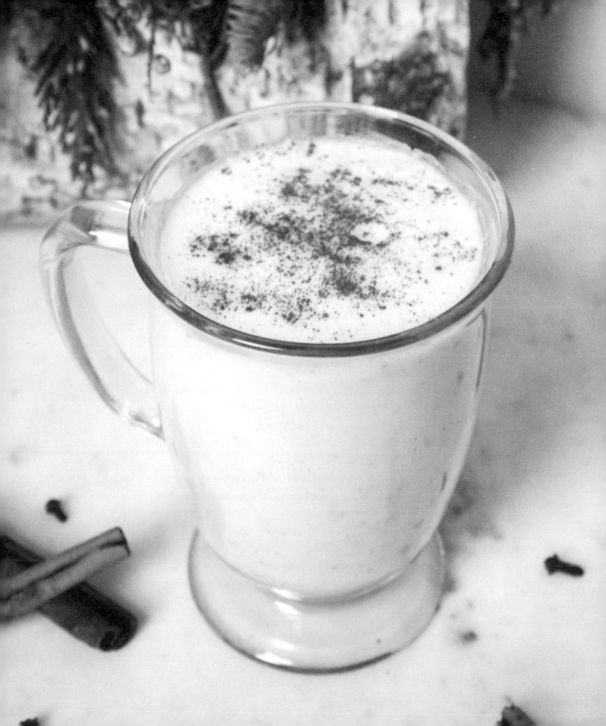

IMPORTANT NUTRIENTS

---◆---

PROTEIN

Alongside fats and carbohydrates, proteins are one of the three main macronutrients. Protein provides structure for cells, regulates the function of tissues and organs, and helps maintain fluid balance. As you can imagine, there is a lot of new cell growth during pregnancy that goes into building a new human, among other things. Eating enough protein is important, particularly since protein comes from the foods you eat and is not found in a prenatal vitamin. During the second and third trimester, protein needs increase by 25 or more grams per day as the baby begins to grow more rapidly. To give you a reference, you could get an extra 25 grams of protein with an extra three-ounce portion of chicken breast or one and a half cups of lentils. Elevated intake should be maintained if you are breastfeeding.

Per the Academy of Nutrition and Dietetics, vegetarian and vegan diets, when well-planned, can meet and even exceed an individual's protein needs. Previously, foods were classified as "complete" or incomplete" depending on whether they provided all of the essential amino acids (those that our bodies cannot make). It was believed that incomplete foods had to be paired, like rice and beans, to reap the benefits. Now, we know that consuming a diverse diet is sufficient for meeting our needs. Eating a variety of plant foods, including legumes and soy, will cover the bases just fine. Consider working with a dietitian to develop a plan that will meet your needs.

VITAMIN A

Vitamin A supports healthy vision as well as normal organ development in a growing child, particularly during the first trimester. Like iron, there are two forms of vitamin A: retinoids (retinol, retinyl esters) derived from animal sources, and provitamin A carotenoids (including beta-carotene) that come from plant foods. Too much or too little vitamin A can have negative effects on a developing child.

Vitamin A deficiency is a common problem in developing parts of the world due to the inaccessability of vitamin A-rich foods. On the contrary, in the U.S. and more developed countries, overconsumption or over-use of vitamin A poses more of a concern. Vitamin A is found in both supplemental and topical form as many medications and creams contain retinol including those to treat acne. Unless directed by your doctor, avoid Vitamin A supplements; instead focus on obtaining the vitamin from your food.

ANIMAL SOURCES (RETINOL): eggs, milk, beef liver

PLANT SOURCES (PROVITAMIN A CAROTENOIDS): spinach, orange and yellow-flesh fruits and vegetables, such as sweet potato, carrots, cantaloupe, mango, oranges, and red peppers

FOLATE

Folate is one of the vitamins that you have probably heard about most in the context of pregnancy. Folate is one of the B vitamins (B9) and is essential for DNA synthesis and cell growth. You may be more familiar with the term "folic acid," the synthetic version that is often added to enriched and fortified products, including breads and cereal, and supplements. Folate is essential for neural tube development, which occurs during the sensitive window when a woman may not know that she is pregnant: for example, within the first month after conception. Having inadequate folate can contribute to neural tube defects, such as spina bifida. Getting the proper amount of folate is important regardless of whether you are trying to become pregnant—as many as 50% of pregnancies are unplanned!

ANIMAL SOURCES: meat, fish, eggs, dairy

PLANT SOURCES: dark leafy greens, beans, avocado, peanuts, tomato, and citrus juice

IRON

Iron is a component of red blood cells that helps shuttle oxygen around the body while promoting normal cell function and the development of connective tissue. During pregnancy, the requirements nearly double to support both the needs of mom and baby. Iron comes in two forms: heme (animal sources) and non-heme (plant sources). Iron absorption, particularly non-heme, is influenced both positively and negatively by other nutrients in foods. For example, pairing vitamin C-rich foods with iron helps the body absorb the mineral. On the other hand, compounds like phytates and tannins, found in coffee and tea, and calcium impair iron absorption.

ANIMAL SOURCES (HEME): fish, beef, poultry

PLANT SOURCES (NON-HEME): beans, lentils, tofu, leafy greens, dried fruits, fortified foods, and dark chocolate

CALCIUM

Calcium is the most abundant mineral in the body. As most of us know, calcium is important for building and maintaining strong bones and teeth, but it also plays critical roles in normal cell function.

ANIMAL SOURCES: dairy, fish with bones (sardines, salmon)

PLANT SOURCES: tofu, leafy greens, and fortified beverages, including orange juice and soy milk

VITAMIN D

Vitamin D plays an important role in helping the body to maintain calcium and phosphorous levels. It acts as a hormone in the body and is unique in that we are able to synthesize vitamin D through sun exposure. Vitamin D is difficult to get from foods, so supplementation may be beneficial in the winter months and/or if you are deficient, which many of us are. Always talk to your doctor before initiating supplements.

ANIMAL SOURCES: salmon (variable depending on the source and type), fortified dairy products, including milk and yogurt, eggs

PLANT SOURCES: fortified products and beverages, such as orange juice and soy milk, and some varieties of mushrooms that have been exposed to UV light (vitamin D2)

VITAMIN B12

Adequate B12, in combination with folate, is important for neurological function and proper development of the nervous system as well as red blood cell formation; in fact, deficiency of B12 can lead to anemia.

ANIMAL SOURCES: widely available; meat, fish, eggs, and cow's milk

PLANT SOURCE: fortified products, such as breakfast cereals, soy milk, and nutritional yeast

ESSENTIAL AND OMEGA-3 FATTY ACIDS

There are certain fats that are "essential" because our body cannot make them. Omega-6 (linoleic acid) and omega-3 (alpha-linolenic acid, ALA) fatty acids both fall under this umbrella. Our bodies can convert ALA to two better-known omega-3 fatty acids—DHA and EPA—but this only occurs in small amounts; thus, consuming foods rich in these fatty acids is necessary. DHA is particularly important in the context of pregnancy and brain development and has been linked to growth outcomes as well as cognitive function in children.

ANIMAL SOURCES: fish, fish oils, and eggs

PLANT SOURCES: nuts, seeds, and microalgae (microalgae is commonly used as a vegan supplement of DHA)

Note: nuts and seeds offer little to no DHA or EPA

CHOLINE

Choline is another essential nutrient that must be obtained through the diet. It serves as a building block for cell membrane components, as well as the neurotransmitter, acetylcholine. In the context of pregnancy, choline plays a crucial role in a normal functioning nervous system and developing brain.

ANIMAL SOURCES: eggs, some cuts of beef, chicken, Atlantic cod

PLANT SOURCES: quinoa, soybeans, beans, and cruciferous vegetables

FOOD SAFETY CONSIDERATIONS DURING PREGNANCY

Food safety isn't the most interesting topic, but it's an important one, particularly during this delicate time. Mom's immune system is suppressed, and baby's immune system is not yet capable of fending for itself. Thus, both are more susceptible to foodborne illness, or food poisoning. Two pathogens that are particularly harmful are *Listeria monocytogenes* and *Toxmoplasma gondii*. To prevent exposure to *Listeria*, always microwave lunch meat and hot dogs before consuming, and avoid refrigerated smoked seafood products, refrigerated pate and meat spreads, and unpasteurized milk products, namely soft cheeses. *Toxmoplasma gondii* can be spread through improper food handling (e.g. not cooking meats to safe internal temperatures or storing improperly, or washing produce with contaminated water), but it can also be spread through contact with contaminated cat litter. If you have a cat, you don't have to get rid of him or her but have someone else maintain the litter box to be safe.

SAFE FOOD HANDLING PRACTICES ACCORDING TO THE FDA

- Always wash hands prior to and after handling food.

- Sanitize kitchen surfaces and keep your refrigerator clean.

- Wash fruits & vegetables. According to a study from the CDC looking at cases of foodborne illness between 1998 and 2008, the majority of reported cases could be attributed to fruits and vegetables, particularly leafy greens. This underscores the importance of washing your produce with clean water—do not use soaps or detergents. Cut off bruises and other damaged spots. Bean sprouts should be avoided, as washing them will not remove harmful bacteria if they got into the seeds prior to growing. Finally, unpasteurized juices, including fresh squeezed juices purchased at farmers markets, restaurants, and juice bars, should be avoided. Note that kombucha is often unpasteurized, which is another reason why we do not promote its consumption during pregnancy.

♦ Safely handle and prepare meat & poultry. The same study from the CDC mentioned above found that 29% of deaths from food-borne illness could be attributed to meat, poultry, pork, and game, with poultry being the biggest culprit (19%). Cook meat, poultry, fish, and eggs to proper internal temperatures and avoid leaving foods out on the counter for extended periods of time. When reheating in the microwave, stir or rotate foods to ensure that cooking is even throughout. Use separate cutting boards and utensils to prepare meats and poultry, and keep these foods contained in the fridge. Never recycle marinades. Store cooked meats in the fridge or freezer.

♦ Choose fish carefully. Avoid raw seafood and types of fish that are high in mercury, including King mackerel, marlin, orange roughy, shark, swordfish, tilefish (from the Gulf of Mexico), and bigeye tuna.

♦ Choose pasteurized dairy and avoid soft cheeses. Store dairy and eggs properly (in the fridge) to prevent growth of pathogens.

♦ Safely store leftovers. Whether from home and or a restaurant, take care to store food in the refrigerator within two hours.

DO I HAVE TO BUY ORGANIC?

This is a controversial topic—surprise, surprise—and the science is mixed. First of all, let's clarify what the term "organic" means. Foods that are labeled organic must meet criteria set by the U.S. Department of Agriculture (USDA). Produce, nuts and seeds, beef, poultry, pork, fish, eggs—all of these foods, and many more, may carry an organic label. For produce, which we will focus on for the purpose of this book, practices that are not allowed in the production of organics include use of synthetic fertilizers, sewage sludge, irradiation, and genetic engineering. Interestingly, this does not exclude use of organic or natural pesticides, insecticides, and fungicides.

Generally speaking, the nutrient composition of organic versus conventional produce is similar, though some differences have been found. For example, organic produce may contain more phytonutrients than conventional produce. More significant differences have been found in studies of animal products: for example, organic milk may have up to 50% more omega 3 fatty acids than conventional. It is worth noting that small amounts of synthetic pesticide residue can be found on organic produce, too. Furthermore, organic does not mean "healthy," and there are plenty of products with an organic label that are energy-dense.

Overall, the consumption of conventional produce comes with an increased risk of exposure to pesticides, and few studies have shown potential health benefits of consuming organic. However, given the state of current evidence, conclusions cannot yet be drawn about the long-term health implications of dietary exposure. Statistically, studying the health effects of consumption of organic versus conventional produce is challenging; one reason for this is that people who purchase organic produce tend to eat differently than people who buy conventional, such that they eat more fruits, vegetables and whole grains, and less meat. However, there is stronger evidence to suggest that occupational exposure to pesticides and chemicals negatively impacts health, including in-utero exposure: i.e. during pregnancy. Researchers from UC Berkeley have been following children born to farmworkers in the Salinas Valley of California for nearly 20 years. This prospective study, called CHAMACOS, has revealed long-term effects of developmental exposure (during pregnancy) to pesticides and chemicals, including but not limited to respiratory and behavioral problems and even differences in the structure of the brain. In 2018, a high-profile case involving Monsanto, maker of an herbicide called Roundup, ruled in favor of a school groundskeeper who claimed that exposure to the weed killer caused his cancer. Thus, there may be other reasons to support organic—and even better, local—farming, including concern for the health and welfare of workers and their families.

When it comes to fruits and vegetables, organic produce may deliver lower levels of pesticides and be a good choice for your pregnancy, but do not let the price tag be a barrier to getting proper nutrition. As the current evidence stands, the benefits of eating a diet rich in plant foods outweigh potential risks related to dietary pesticide exposure. If you are concerned, here are some suggestions for minimizing pesticide exposure: wash fruits and vegetables thoroughly, dry them with a paper towel, and pick off outer leaves.

STRATEGIES FOR ORDERING HEALTHY MOCKTAILS WHEN DINING OUT

- **Avoid sodas and tonic water.** Choose unsweetened seltzer instead.

- **Avoid drink mixes** (e.g. margarita mix) and creamy, frozen, and "-ade" drinks. These are calorie and sugar bombs!

- **Add a splash of juice to seltzer or water for flavor but avoid fresh squeezed juices and juice cocktails.** Or, cut juice with seltzer water (50/50) to decrease the sugar content. While all juices have something to offer in the way of nutrients, pomegranate and 100% cranberry juice are particularly high in antioxidants.

- **Choose unsweetened teas over sweetened but watch the quantity if you aren't drinking decaf.**

- **Infuse flavor in drinks by asking for herbs, spices (like cinnamon), or pieces of fresh fruit, like lemon, lime or orange.**

- **Ask the bartender to transform your favorite traditional drinks into alcohol-free and low sugar versions.** Mojitos, margaritas, and Bloody Marys, to name a few, can be easily made without the addition of alcohol. Instead of sugar, ask for your drink to be made with a small amount of flavored or infused simple syrup (less than half a fluid ounce or one tablespoon). A little can go a long way, especially for strong flavors, like ginger.

RELIABLE RESOURCES FOR PREGNANCY, NUTRITION, AND HEALTH

In this section, we provide a list of resources and organizations that informed the development of this book and that we believe are "reputable." This list is by no means exhaustive. Please keep in mind that consulting even the most reliable sources on the web is not a replacement for talking to your doctor and seeking individualized medical advice.

BOOKS ON NUTRITION & PREGNANCY FROM REGISTERED DIETITIANS AND OTHER CREDENTIALED PROFESSIONALS

◆ *Expect the Best: Your Guide to Eating Healthy Before, During and After Pregnancy, Second Edition*
Written by Elizabeth Ward, an RDN, LDN, this book is approved by the Academy of Nutrition and Dietetics. It is a comprehensive but approachable resource for women, providing recipes and guidance for nutrition from the preconception to postpartum phases. We heavily referenced this book in Chapter 1!

◆ *What to Eat When You're Pregnant: A Week-by-Week Guide to Support Your Health and Your Baby's Development*
Written by neuroscientist Dr. Nicole Avena (PhD), this book provides evidenced-base recommendations and recipes for how to eat when you're pregnant. Dr. Avena (also co-author of the book *Why Diets Fail: Science Explains How to End Cravings, Lose Weight, and Get Healthy*) has a very balanced approach.

- *Real Food For Pregnancy: The Science and Wisdom of Optimal Prenatal Nutrition (& Real Food For Gestational Diabetes)*
  Written by Lily Nichols, RDN and founder of pilatesnutritionist.com. Lily advocates a real food approach that translates into a lower-carb diet. While her perspective is somewhat controversial and sometimes even at odds with the recommendations of the Academy of Nutrition and Dietetics, the evidence that she presents is compelling.

- *The Fertility Diet: Groundbreaking Research Reveals Natural Ways to Boost Ovulation and Improve Your Chances of Getting Pregnant*
  Written by Harvard researchers, this book translates evidence from the Nurses' Health Study, a long-running prospective cohort study, into guidance for women who are trying to improve their chances of conceiving.

- *The Whole 9 Months: A Week-By-Week Pregnancy Nutrition Guide with Recipes for a Healthy Start*
  Written by Jennifer Lang, MD and Dana Angelo White, MS, RD, this book contains whole food, plant-based recipes for your pregnancy developed by a Registered Dietitian with guidance written by both authors.

- *Fertility Foods Cookbook: 100+ Recipes to Nourish Your Body*
  Written by Elizabeth Shaw, RDN and Sara Haas, RDN, this book provides fresh perspective with nutrition guidance and recipes for those trying or struggling to conceive.

- *The Predominantly Plant-Based Pregnancy Guide*
  Alex Caspero, MA, RDN, and Whitney English Tabaie, MS, RDN, provide evidence-based information on everything that the plant-based mom-to-be needs to know to have a healthy pregnancy. This book includes 50+ recipes as well as exercise and lifestyle tips. https://plantbasedjuniors.lpages.co/pregnancy-guide-full/

REPUTABLE ORGANIZATIONS

- Academy of Nutrition and Dietetics
- American College of Obstetricians and Gynecologists
- American Academy of Pediatrics
- American College of Nurse-Midwives
- National Institute on Alcohol Abuse and Alcoholism
- National Organization on Fetal Alcohol Spectrum Disorders
- March of Dimes
- National Institute of Child Health and Development
- Centers for Disease Control and Prevention
- Food and Drug Administration
- U.S. Department of Agriculture

ADDITIONAL ONLINE RESOURCES FOR NUTRITION, HEALTH, AND PREGNANCY CAN BE FOUND AT:

DIANALICALZI.COM/DRINKINGFORTWO

The following publications provided background information that informed the book.

Avena, N. (2015). *What to Eat When You're Pregnant: A Week-by-Week Guide to Support Your Health and Your Baby's Development.* Berkeley, CA: Ten Speed Press

Chavarro, J., Willett, W., Skerrett, P. (2009). *The Fertility Diet: Groundbreaking Research Reveals Natural Ways to Boost Ovulation and Improve Your Chances of Getting Pregnant.* New York, NY: McGraw-Hill Education

Nichols, L. (2018). *Real Food for Pregnancy: The Science and Wisdom of Optimal Prenatal Nutrition.* Publisher: Author

Ward, E. (2009) *Expect the Best: Your Guide to Healthy Eating Before, During, and After Pregnancy.* Nashville, TN: Turner Publishing Company

CHAPTER 1

NUTRITION PRIMER

"Given the innumerable health benefits of consuming these foods" (Page 14) : Slavin, L., J., Beate, & Lloyd. (2012). Health Benefits of Fruits and Vegetables. *Advances in Nutrition, 3*(4), 506-516. https://doi.org/10.3945/an.112.002154

"Also, be mindful that "wheat flour" is different than whole wheat flour." (Page 14) : Elkus, G. (n.d.). The Difference Between Whole Wheat, Whole Grain, and Multigrain Bread. Retrieved from https://www.realsimple.com/food-recipes/cooking-tips-techniques/whole-wheat-whole-grain-breads-0

"According to the Academy of Nutrition and Dietetics" (Page 14) : Melina, V., Craig, W., Levin, S.

(2016) Position of the Academy of Nutrition and Dietetics: Vegetarian Diets. *Journal of the Academy of Nutrition and Dietetics, 116*(12), 1970-1980. https://doi.org/10.1016/j.jand.2016.09.025

"Plant-based diets have numerous health benefits" (Page 14) : Nelson, M. E., Hamm, M. W., Hu, F. B., Abrams, S. A., & Griffin, T. S. (2016). Alignment of Healthy Dietary Patterns and Environmental Sustainability: A Systematic Review. *Advances in Nutrition, 7*(6), 1005-1025. https://doi.org/10.3945/an.116.012567

"In the context of pregnancy, numerous studies have demonstrated" (Page 15) : Pistollato, F., Cano, S. S., Elio, I., Vergara, M. M., Giampieri, F., & Battino, M. (2015). Plant-Based and Plant-Rich Diet Patterns during Gestation: Beneficial Effects and Possible Shortcomings. *Advances in Nutrition, 6*(5), 581-591. https://doi.org/10.3945/an.115.009126

"as consumption has been linked to increased risk of death and chronic disease" (Page 15) : Schwingshackl, L., Schwedhelm, C., Hoffmann, G. (2017). Food groups and risk of all-cause mortality: a systematic review and meta-analysis of prospective studies. *The American Journal of Clinical Nutrition, 105*(6), 1462–73. https://doi.org/10.3945/ajcn.117.153148

"For example, in a 2015 update to a previous report, the World Cancer Research Fund" (Page 15) : Vieira, A., Abar, L., Chan, D., Stevens, C., Polemiti, E., Greenwood, D., & Norat, T. (2017). Foods and beverages and colorectal cancer risk: A systematic review and meta-analysis of cohort studies, an update of the evidence of the WCRF-AICR Continuous Update Project. *Annals of Oncology, 28*(8), 1788–1802. https://doi.org/10.1093/annonc/mdx171

"The 2015-2020 Dietary Guidelines for Americans" (Page 16) : U.S. Department of Health and Human Services and U.S. Department of Agriculture. 2015–2020 Dietary Guidelines for Americans. 8th Edition.

December 2015. Available at http://health.gov/dietaryguidelines/2015/guidelines/.

"the type of fat that has been linked to cardiovascular disease" (Page 16) : Sacks, F., Lichtenstein, A., Wu, J., Appel, L., Creager, M., et al. (2017). Dietary Fats and Cardiovascular Disease: A Presidential Advisory From the American Heart Association. *Circulation, 136*, e1-e23. http://doi.org/10.1161/CIR.0000000000000510

"may be beneficial in the context of fertility" (Page 16) : Chavarro, J., Willett, W., Skerrett, P. (2009). *The Fertility Diet: Groundbreaking Research Reveals Natural Ways to Boost Ovulation and Improve Your Chances of Getting Pregnant.* New York, NY: McGraw-Hill Education

"Each of the non-dairy milk options offers unique flavors, textures, and nutrient profiles" (Page 16) : Drayer, L. (2018, May 31). Got alt-milk? Retrieved from https://www.cnn.com/2018/05/31/health/alternative-milk-food-drayer/index.html

"including close to ½ of the protein content of the whole egg." (Page 16) : Huizen, J. (2017, December 27). Egg yolk: Nutrition and benefits. Retrieved from https://www.medicalnewstoday.com/articles/320445.php

"the 2015-2020 Dietary Guidelines" (Page 16) : U.S. Department of Health and Human Services and U.S. Department of Agriculture. 2015–2020 Dietary Guidelines for Americans. 8th Edition. December 2015. Available at http://health.gov/dietaryguidelines/2015/guidelines/.

"did not include cholesterol as a nutrient for concern" (Page 17) : Skerrett, P. J. (2015, February 12). Panel suggests that dietary guidelines stop warning about cholesterol in food. Retrieved from https://www.health.harvard.edu/blog/panel-suggests-stop-warning-about-cholesterol-in-food-201502127713

"A meta-analysis published in 2015

found that dietary cholesterol was not associated" (Page 17) : Berger, S., Raman, G., Vishwanathan, R., Jacques, P., & Johnson, E. (2015). Dietary cholesterol and cardiovascular disease: A systematic review and meta-analysis. *The American Journal of Clinical Nutrition, 102*(2), 276–294. https://doi.org/10.3945/ajcn.114.100305

"many women are at risk for excessive weight gain" (Page 17) : Catalano, P., Shankar, K. (2016). Obesity and pregnancy: mechanisms of short term and long term adverse consequences for mother and child. *BMJ, 360*, j1. https://doi.org/10.1136/bmj.j1

"According to the 2009 guidelines set forth by the Institute of Medicine, women within a "normal" range for weight prior to pregnancy should expect to gain 25-35 lbs during pregnancy." (Page 17) : Institute of Medicine (US) and National Research Council (US) Committee to Reexamine IOM Pregnancy Weight Guidelines; Rasmussen KM, Yaktine AL, editors (2009). *Weight Gain During Pregnancy: Reexamining the Guidelines.* Washington (DC): National Academies Press (US).

"The Academy of Nutrition and Dietetics recommends that pregnant women consume three liters" (Page 18) : Kaiser, L., Campbell, C. (2014). Nutrition and LIfestyle for a Healthy Pregnancy Outcome. *Academy of Nutrition and Dietetics, 114*(9). Retrieved from: https://www.eatrightpro.org/-/media/eatrightpro-files/practice/position-and-practice-papers/practice-papers/practice_paper_healthy_pregnancy.df?la=en&hash=D957510D25115813BD792F92D996B945FD07D4B8

"Alcohol use and abuse is on the rise in the United States. A study published in 2017 revealed" (Page 18) : Grant, B., Chou, S., Saha, T., Pickering, R., et al. (2017). Prevalence of 12-Month Alcohol Use, High-Risk Drinking, and DSM-IV Alcohol Use Disorder in the United States, 2001-2002 to 2012-2013. *JAMA Psychiatry,*

74(9), 911-923. http://doi.org/10.1001/jamapsychiatry.2017.2161

"However, recent evidence suggests that the current guidelines for alcohol consumption may be too lenient." (Page 18) : Wood, A., Kaptoge, S., Butterworth, A., Willeit S., Warnakula S., et al. (2018). Risk thresholds for alcohol consumption: combined analysis of individual-participant data for 599 912 current drinkers in 83 prospective studies. *The Lancet, 391*, 1513-1523. https://doi.org/10.1016/S0140-6736(18)30134-X

"For reference, the recommended upper limit..." (Page 19) : Kalinowski, A., and Humphreys, K. (2016) Governmental standard drink definitions and low-risk alcohol consumption guidelines in 37 countries. Addiction, 111: 1293–1298. doi: 10.1111/add.13341.

"1 standard drink = 14 grams pure alcohol" (Page 19) : What is A Standard Drink? (n.d.) Retrieved from https://www.niaaa.nih.gov/alcohol-health/overview-alcohol-consumption/what-standard-drink

"For example, a 2015 analysis examining prospective data of women (and men) enrolled in the Health Professionals Study" (Page 19) : Cao, Y., Willett, W., Rimm, E., Stampfer, M., Giovannucci, E. (2015). Light to moderate intake of alcohol, drinking patterns, and risk of cancer: results from two prospective US cohort studies. *BMJ, 351*, h4238. http://doi.org/10.1136/bmj.h4238

"Alcohol and Pregnancy" (Page 19) : Nawaz, A., (2018, July 28): Fetal alcohol disorders are more common than you think. Retrieved from https://www.pbs.org/newshour/show/fetal-alcohol-disorder-is-more-common-than-you-think

"According to a study published by the CDC in 2015" (Page 19) : as summarized in Key Findings: Alcohol use and binge drinking among women of childbearing age – United States, 2011-2013 (2018, July 31). Retrieved from http://www.cdc.gov/ncbddd/fasd/features/drinking-childbearing-age.html

"a statement that is supported by the CDC" (Page 20) : Alcohol Use in Pregnancy. (2018, July 17). Retrieved from https://www.cdc.gov/ncbddd/

fasd/alcohol-use.html

"U.S. Surgeon General" (Page 20) : Notice to Readers: Surgeon General's Advisory on Alcohol Use in Pregnancy. (2005, March 11). Retrieved from: https://www.cdc.gov/mmwr/preview/mmwrhtml/mm5409a6.htm

"American Academy of Pediatrics" (Page 20) : AAP Says No Amount of Alcohol Should be Considered Safe During Pregnancy. (2015, October 19). Retrieved from https://www.aap.org/en-us/about-the-aap/aap-press-room/Pages/AAP-Says-No-Amount-of-Alcohol-Should-be-Considered-Safe-During-Pregnancy.aspx

"A study released in 2018 updated the statistics on prevalence" (Page 20) : May, P., Chambers, C., Kalberg, W., Zellner, J., et.al. (2018). Prevalence of Fetal Alcohol Spectrum Disorders in 4 US Communities. *JAMA, 319(5)*, 474-482. http://doi.org/10.1001/jama.2017.21896

"some doctors even tell their patients that one drink probably won't hurt." (Page 21) : Is it safe for a woman to have an occasional beer, glass of wine, or other alcoholic beverage when she is pregnant? (n.d.). Retrieved from https://www.nofas.org/light-drinking/

"But, as Dr. Michael Charness points out, when it comes to the controversy surrounding drinking while pregnant" (Page 21) : Is it safe for a woman to have an occasional beer, glass of wine, or other alcoholic beverage when she is pregnant? (n.d.). Retrieved from https://www.nofas.org/light-drinking/

"that roughly 45% of pregnancies are unplanned, and a woman may not know she is pregnant for several weeks." (Page 21) : Finka, L., Zolna, M. (2016). Declines in Unintended Pregnancy in the United States, 2008-2011. *The New England Journal of Medicine, 374*, 843-52. http://doi.org/10.1056/NEJMsa1506575

"and there is an ongoing debate over whether to label kombucha" (Page 22) : Wyatt, K. (2015, October 12). As kombucha sales boom, makers ask feds for new alcohol test. Retrieved from https://www.coloradoan.com/story/news/2015/10/12/kombucha-sales-boom-makers-ask-feds-new-alcohol-test/73848710/

"whether to label kombucha as an alcoholic beverage." (Page 22) : Kombucha Information and Resources. (n.d.). Retrieved from https://www.ttb.gov/kombucha/kombucha-general.shtml

"This prompted some brands to take action and start independently verifying the alcohol content of their kombucha." (Page 22) : Pomranz, M. (2017, June 22). The Hot Debate Over Kombucha's Alcohol Content. Retrieved from https://www.foodandwine.com/fwx/drink/hot-debate-over-kombucha-s-alcohol-content

"it may be difficult to know beyond a reasonable doubt how much alcohol is actually in these drinks" (Page 22) : Hamblin, J. (2016, December 8). Is Fermented Tea Making People Feel Enlightened Because of ... Alcohol? Retrieved from: https://www.theatlantic.com/health/archive/2016/12/the-promises-of-kombucha/509786/

"Furthermore, most kombuchas are raw, meaning not pasteurized" (Page 22) : Kombucha: The Best and Worst Brands. (n.d.). Retrieved from https://healthyeater.com/healthiest-kombucha-brands

"For someone consuming 2,000 calories a day, this is less than 200 calories from added sugars, or 50 grams per day." (Page 22) : Cut Down on Added Sugars. (2016, March). Retrieved from https://health.gov/dietaryguidelines/2015/resources/DGA_Cut-Down-On-Added-Sugars.pdf

"anhydrous dextrose, brown sugar, confectioner's powdered sugar..." (Page 23) : What are added sugars? (2016, November 6). Retrieved from https://www.choosemyplate.gov/what-are-added-sugars

"In fact, the WHO classifies juice" (Page 23) : World Health Organization. (2015). *Guideline: Sugars intake for adults and children*. United States: World Health Organization. Retrieved from: http://apps.who.int/iris/bitstream/handle/10665/149782/9789241549028_eng.pdf%3Bjsessionid=FDC81E9F441FFE745B9A5924B91135ED?sequence=1

"the only consistent conclusion is that more research is needed." (Page 24) : Auerbach, B., Dibey, S., Vallila-Buchman, P., et al. (2018). Review of 100% Fruit Juice and Chronic Health Conditions: Implications for Sugar-Sweetened Beverage Policy. *Advances in Nutrition, 9(2)*, 78–85. https://doi.org/10.1093/advances/nmx006

"The current recommendations of the Dietary Guidelines for Americans" (Page 24) : U.S. Department of Health and Human Services and U.S. Department of Agriculture. 2015–2020 Dietary Guidelines for Americans. 8th Edition. December 2015. Available at http://health.gov/dietaryguidelines/2015/guidelines/.

"What's more, you are saving quite a few calories by removing the alcohol itself, 7 calories per gram" (Page 24) : Hilton Anderson, C. (2015, May 4). The Calorie Count of All Your Favorite Cocktails. Retrieved from https://www.shape.com/healthy-eating/healthy-drinks/calorie-count-all-your-favorite-cocktails

"Some evidence suggests that chemical sweeteners may impact blood glucose levels by altering insulin release" (Page 25) : Mattes, R., Popkin, B. (2009). Nonnutritive sweetener consumption in humans: effects on appetite and food intake and their putative mechanisms. *American Journal of Clinical Nutrition, 89(1)*, 1-14. https://doi.org/10.3945/ajcn.2008.26792

"the gut microbiome." (Page 25) : Suez, J., Korem, T., Zilberman-Schapira, G., Segal, E., Elinav, F. (2015). Non-caloric artificial sweeteners and the microbiome: findings and challenges. *Gut Microbes, 6(2)*, 149-155. http://doi.org/10.1080/19490976.2015.1017700

"In addition, a Canadian cohort study published in 2016 revealed that children born" (Page 25) : Azad, M., Sharma, A., de Souza, R., et al. (2016). Association Between Artificially Sweetened Beverage Consumption During Pregnancy and Infant Body Mass Index. *JAMA Pediatrics, 170(7)*, 662-670. http://doi.org/10.1001/jamapediatrics.2016.0301

"Caffeine." (Page 25) : Caffeine in Pregnancy. (2015, October). Retrieved from https://www.marchofdimes.org/pregnancy/caffeine-in-pregnancy.aspx

"Consumption above this recommended threshold increases the risk of miscarriage among other complications." (Page 26) : Weng, X., Odouli, R., De-Kun, Li. (2008). Maternal caffeine consumption during pregnancy and the risk of miscarriage: a prospective cohort study. *American Journal of Obstetrics and Gynecology*, 198, 279.e1-279.e8. http://doi.org/10.1016/j.ajog.2007.10.803

"A recent study from Norway observed an association between caffeine consumption during pregnancy" (Page 26) : Papadopoulou E., Botton J., Brantsæter A-L., et al. (2018). Maternal caffeine intake during pregnancy and childhood growth and overweight: results from a large Norwegian prospective observational cohort study. *BMJ Open*, 8, e018895. http://doi.org/10.1136/bmjopen-2017-018895

"The Food and Drug Administration (FDA) only reviews the safety of ingredients" (Page 26) : Dietary Supplements: What You Need to Know. (2017, November 29). Retrieved from https://www.fda.gov/Food/DietarySupplements/UsingDietarySupplements/ucm109760.htm

"Use caution when brewing yourself herbal teas, as some contain ingredients that may not be safe for consumption" (Page 27) : Herbal Tea and Pregnancy. (2018, October 8). Retrieved from http://americanpregnancy.org/pregnancy-health/herbal-tea/

"You can also steep fruit, peels, or spices" (Page 27) : Herbal Remedies, Supplements and Teas During Pregnancy. (2018, October 14). Retrieved from https://www.whattoexpect.com/pregnancy/eating-well/week-19/natural-woman.aspx

"Red raspberry leaf tea is often promoted" (Page 27) : Raspberry Leaf 101. (2015, July 7). Retrieved from https://www.traditionalmedicinals.com/articles/plants/raspberry-leaf-101/

As many as 75% of women experience nausea and/or vomiting" (Page 28) : Lee, N., Saha, S. (2011). Nausea and Vomiting of Pregnancy.

Gastroenterology Clinics of North America, 40(2). 309–334. http://doi.org/10.1016/j.gtc.2011.03.009

"According to the Academy of Nutrition and Dietetics, the most common food aversions are to coffee, tea, fried or fatty foods, highly spiced foods, meat, and eggs." (Page 28) : Kaiser, L., Campbell, C. (2014). Nutrition and LIfestyle for a Healthy Pregnancy Outcome. *Academy of Nutrition and Dietetics*, 114(9). Retrieved from https://www.eatrightpro.org/-/media/eatrightpro-files/practice/position-and-practice-papers/practice-papers/practice_paper_healthy_pregnancy.pdf?la=en&hash=D957510D25115813BD792F92D996B945FD07D4B8

"as they can suppress our feelings of fullness" (Page 29) : Avena, N. (2015). *What to Eat When You're Pregnant: A Week-by-Week Guide to Support Your Health and Your Baby's Development.* Berkeley, CA: Ten Speed Press

"Common food cravings during pregnancy include chocolate, citrus fruits, pickles, chips, and ice cream" (Page 29) : Avena, N. (2015). *What to Eat When You're Pregnant: A Week-by-Week Guide to Support Your Health and Your Baby's Development.* Berkeley, CA: Ten Speed Press

"Cravings for sweets tend to peak mid-gestation." (Page 29) : Avena, N. (2015). *What to Eat When You're Pregnant: A Week-by-Week Guide to Support Your Health and Your Baby's Development.* Berkeley, CA: Ten Speed Press

"Having someone else prepare food or drinks for you may also be helpful with sensitivities to smells." (Page 30) : Nichols, L. (2018). *Real Food for Pregnancy: The Science and Wisdom of Optimal Prenatal Nutrition.* Publisher: Author

"Reflux" (Page 30) : Johnson, A. (2018, June 7). Gastroesophageal Reflux. Retrieved from https://www.eatright.org/health/wellness/digestive-health/gastroesophageal-reflux

"This can happen at any time during pregnancy but is more common during the third trimester." (Page 30) : Avena, N. (2015). *What to Eat When You're Pregnant: A Week-by-Week Guide to Support Your Health and Your Baby's Development.* Berkeley, CA:

Ten Speed Press

"Getting enough potassium is also important" (Page 31) : (2009, April). Potassium and Sodium out of Balance. Retrieved from https://www.health.harvard.edu/newsletter_article/Potassium_and_sodium_out_of_balance

"Gestational diabetes" (Page 31) : Diabetes Management Guidelines. (n.d.). Retrieved from http://www.ndei.org/ADA-diabetes-management-guidelines-diabetes-in-pregnancy-GDM.aspx.html

"developing child as well as the mother and may impact as many as 18% of pregnancies" (Page 31) : Visser GH, de Valk HW. (2013). Is the evidence strong enough to change the diagnostic criteria for gestational diabetes now? *American Journal of Obstetrics and Gynecology*, 208(4), 260–264. http://doi.org/10.1016/j.ajog.2012.10.881

"women who develop GDM have a higher risk—35-60%—of developing Type II diabetes" (Page 31) : Bellamy, L., Casa, J.P., Hingorani A., Williams, D. (2009) Type 2 diabetes mellitus after gestational diabetes: a systematic review and meta-analysis. *The Lancet*, 373, 1773–79. https://doi.org/10.1016/S0140-6736(09)60731-5

"Be sure not to restrict sodium intake below the Dietary Guidelines" (Page 32) : U.S. Department of Health and Human Services and U.S. Department of Agriculture. 2015–2020 Dietary Guidelines for Americans. 8th Edition. December 2015. Available at http://health.gov/dietaryguidelines/2015/guidelines/.

"A prospective study in Canada examining the relationship between prepregnancy BMI and maternal and infant outcomes" (Page 32) : Schummers, L., Hutcheon, J., Bodnar, L., et al. (2015) Risk of Adverse Pregnancy Outcomes by Prepregnancy Body Mass Index: A Population-Based Study to Inform Prepregnancy Weight Loss Counseling. *Obstetrics & Gynecology*, 125(1), 133–143. http://doi.org/10.1097/AOG.0000000000000591

"Moderate caffeine and alcohol consumption prior to pregnancy" (Page 34) : Gaskins, A., Chavarro,

J. (2018) Diet and fertility: a review. *American Journal of Obstetrics & Gynecology*, 218(4), 379-389. https://doi.org/10.1016/j.ajog.2017.08.010

"alcohol in particular certainly will not help you get pregnant." (Page 34) : Chavarro, J., Willett, W., Skerrett, P. (2009). *The Fertility Diet: Groundbreaking Research Reveals Natural Ways to Boost Ovulation and Improve Your Chances of Getting Pregnant.* New York, NY: McGraw-Hill Education

"Postpartum" (Page 34) : Cait's Plate. (2018, April 11). Nutrition After Pregnancy for Nursing Mothers. [blog post]. Retrieved from https://caitsplate.com/nutrition-after-pregnancy-for-nursing-mothers/

"unexpected outcomes of labor and delivery that result in significant short- or long-term consequences to a women's health." (Page 34) : Severe Maternal Morbidity in the United States. (n.d.). Retrieved from https://www.cdc.gov/reproductivehealth/maternalinfanthealth/severematernalmorbidity.html

"in fact, an American woman has three times the risk of dying relative to a woman from Canada" (Page 35) : Martin, N. and Anderson, M. (2018, May 10). Retrieved from https://www.npr.org/2018/05/10/607782992/for-every-woman-who-dies-in-childbirth-in-the-u-s-70-more-come-close

"a supplement may be indicated if you do not consume these foods." (Page 35) : Ward, E. (2009) *Expect the Best: Your Guide to Healthy Eating Before, During, and After Pregnancy.* Nashville, TN: Turner Publishing Company

"significantly reduced the risk of having a baby with a higher than desired birth weight" (Page 36) : Jain AP, Gavard JA, Rice JJ, et al. (2012). The impact of interpregnancy weight change on birthweight in obese women. *American Journal of Obstetrics & Gynecology*, 208, 205.e1-7. https://doi.org/10.1016/j.ajog.2012.12.018

"may consume alcohol in moderation but should allow at least two hours before pumping" (Page 36) : Eidelman, A., Schanler, R. (2012). Breastfeeding and the Use of Human

REFERENCES

Milk. *Pediatrics, 129* (3), e827. http://doi.org/10.1542/peds.2011-3552

"impairing your ability to breastfeed while it is active in your system." (Page 36) : Ward, E. (2009) *Expect the Best: Your Guide to Healthy Eating Before, During, and After Pregnancy.* Nashville, TN: Turner Publishing Company

"For example, higher weight and poor diet quality (i.e. an energy-dense diet) have both been associated" (Page 36) : Stephenson, J., Heslehurst, N., Hall, J., et. al. (2018). Before the beginning: nutrition and lifestyle in the preconception period and its importance for future health. *The Lancet, 391,* 1830–41. http://dx.doi.org/10.1016/S0140-6736(18)30311-8

APPENDIX 1
IMPORTANT NUTRIENTS

"During the second and third trimester, protein needs increase by 25 or more grams per day" (Page 144) : Ward, E. (2009) *Expect the Best: Your Guide to Healthy Eating Before, During, and After Pregnancy.* Nashville, TN: Turner Publishing Company

"as the baby begins to grow more rapidly." (Page 144) : Cait's Plate. (2018, March 30). The Role of Nutrition During Pregnancy. [blog post]. Retrieved from https://caitsplate.com/the-role-of-nutrition-during-pregnancy/

"Academy of Nutrition and Dietetics" (Page 144) : Melina, V., Craig, W., Levin, S. (2016). Position of the Academy of Nutrition and Dietetics: Vegetarian Diets. *Journal of the Academy of Nutrition and Dietetics, 116*(12), 1970-1980. https://doi.org/10.1016/j.jand.2016.09.025

"Now, we know that consuming a diverse diet is sufficient for meeting our needs" (Page 144) : Greger, M. (2015, April 25). The Protein-Combining Myth. Retrieved from https://nutritionfacts.org/video/the-protein-combining-myth/

"Vitamin A" (Page 145) : Vitamin A: Fact Sheet for Health Professionals. (2018, October 5). Retrieved from https://ods.od.nih.gov/factsheets/VitaminA-HealthProfessional/

"Folate" (Page 145) : Folate: Fact Sheet for Health Professionals. (2018, October 4). Retrieved from https://ods.od.nih.gov/factsheets/Folate-HealthProfessional/

"Iron" (Page 146) : Iron: Fact Sheet for Health Professionals. (2018, December 7). Retrieved from https://ods.od.nih.gov/factsheets/Iron-HealthProfessional/

"Calcium" (Page 146) : Calcium: Fact Sheet for Health Professionals. (2018, December 7). Retrieved from https://ods.od.nih.gov/factsheets/Iron-Health-Professional/

"Vitamin D" (Page 146) : Vitamin D: Fact Sheet for Health Professionals. (2018, November 9). Retrieved from https://ods.od.nih.gov/factsheets/VitaminD-HealthProfessional/

"some varieties of mushrooms that have been exposed to UV light" (Page 146) : Greger, M. (2013, August 1). Vitamin D from Mushrooms, Sun, or Supplements? Retrieved from https://nutritionfacts.org/2013/08/01/vitamin-d-from-mushrooms-sun-or-supplements/

"Vitamin B12" (Page 147) : Vitamin B12: Fact Sheet for Health Professionals. (2018, November 29). Retrieved from: https://ods.od.nih.gov/factsheets/VitaminB12-HealthProfessional/

"Essential and Omega 3 fatty acids" (Page 147) : Cait's Plate. (2018, March 30). The Role of Nutrition During Pregnancy. [blog post]. Retrieved from https://caitsplate.com/the-role-of-nutrition-during-pregnancy/

"Choline" (Page 147) : Choline: Fact Sheet for Health Professionals. (2018, September 26). Retrieved from https://ods.od.nih.gov/factsheets/Choline-Health-Professional/

APPENDIX 2
FOOD SAFETY CONSIDERATIONS

"Food safety considerations" (Page 148) : Food Safety for Pregnant Women. (2011, September). Retrieved from https://www.fda.gov/food/foodborneillnesscontaminants/peopleatrisk/ucm312704.htm

"To prevent exposure to Listeria" (Page 148) : Listeria and Pregnancy. (2018, June). Retrieved from https://www.acog.org/Patients/FAQs/Listeria-and-Pregnancy?IsMobileSet=false

"*Toxmoplasma gondii* can be spread through improper food handling" (Page 148) : Parasites-Toxoplasmosis (Toxoplasma Infection). (n.d.). Retrieved from https://www.cdc.gov/parasites/toxoplasmosis/gen_info/pregnant.html

"food pulled from the FDA's website" (Page 148) : Food Safety for Moms to Be. (n.d.). Retrieved from https://www.fda.gov/Food/FoodborneIllnessContaminants/PeopleAtRisk/ucm081785.htm

"According to a study from the CDC" (Page 148) : Attribution of Foodborne Illness: Findings. (n.d.).

Retrieved from https://www.cdc.gov/foodborneburden/attribution/attribution-1998-2008.html

APPENDIX 3
DO I HAVE TO BUY ORGANIC?

"Interestingly, this does not exclude use of organic or natural pesticides, insecticides, and fungicides." (Page 150) : About Organic Produce. (n.d.). Retrieved from https://www.ocf.berkeley.edu/~lhom/organictext.html

"the nutrient composition of organic versus conventional produce is similar" (Page 150) : Mie, A., Andersen, H., Gunnarsson, S., et al. (2017). Human health implications of organic food and organic agriculture: a comprehensive review. *Environmental Health, 16*(111). https://doi.org/10.1186/s12940-017-0315-4

"with an increased risk of exposure to pesticides" (Page 150) : Freinkel, S. (2014, March 11). Warning Signs: How Pesticides Harm the Young Brain. Retrieved from https://www.thenation.com/article/warning-signs-how-pesticides-harm-young-brain/

"conclusions cannot yet be drawn about the long-term health implications of dietary exposure" (Page 150) : Smith-Spangler, C., Brandeau, M., Hunter, G., et al. (2012). Are organic foods safer or healthier than conventional alternatives? A systematic review. *Annals of Internal Medicine, 157*(5), 348-66. http://doi.org/10.7326/0003-4819-157-5-201209040-00007

"one reason for this is that people who purchase organic produce" (Page 150) : Mie, A., Andersen, H., Gunnarsson, S., et al. (2017). Human health implications of organic food and organic agriculture: a comprehensive review. *Environmental Health, 16*(111). https://doi.org/10.1186/s12940-017-0315-4

"This prospective study, called CHAMACOS" (Page 151) : CHAMACOS Study. (n.d.). Retrieved from https://cerch.berkeley.edu/research-programs/chamacos-study

"In 2018, a high-profile case involving Monsanto" (Page 151) : Wamsley, L. (2018, October 23). California Judge Cuts Award To $78.5 Million In Monsanto Weedkiller Case. Retrieved from https://www.npr.org/2018/10/23/659848853/california-judge-cuts-award-to-78-5-million-in-monsanto-weedkiller-case

ABOUT THE AUTHORS

KERRY BENSON, MS, RD is a registered dietitian and holds a master's degree in Nutritional Epidemiology from Tufts University. Prior to becoming a dietitian, she earned a master's degree in Behavioral Neuroscience and worked in a research lab for more than six years studying the effects of alcohol exposure during pregnancy on the developing brain. This experience sparked her interest in the topic of drinking, particularly in the context of pregnancy. She is a licensed dietitian in the state of Pennsylvania. She enjoys photography, staying active, tending to her plants, and, of course, cooking.

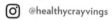 @healthycrayvings

DIANA LICALZI MALDONADO, MS, RD is a registered dietitian and holds a master's degree in Nutrition Science and Policy from Tufts Friedman School of Nutrition Science and Policy. Originally from Puerto Rico, Diana is dedicated to helping the Hispanic community meet their nutrition and health goals. She co-founded Reversing T2D, an online platform that provides nutritional guidance for individuals with pre- and type 2 diabetes. Diana also has experience working as a Dietitian at Boston Medical Center, InsideTracker, and UC San Diego Health. You'll often find Diana outside—running, hiking, or practicing yoga—or experimenting in the kitchen.

@dietitian.diana